TABLE OF CONTENTS

3 INTRODUCTION
- What Is WW? — 3
- How does Weigh Watchers work? — 4
- Will WW help you lose weight ? — 5
- Shopping Guide — 6

8 BREAKFAST
- Blueberry French Toast Casserole — 9
- Homemade Cinnamon Roll Recipe — 10
- Tater Tot Breakfast Casserole — 11
- Sausage Breakfast CasseroleOmelet — 12
- Fluffy Homemade Waffle — 13
- Chorizo Breakfast Hash — 14
- Homemade Shredded Hashbrowns — 15

16 SOUP
- Coconut Curry Soup — 17
- Minestrone Soup — 18
- Chicken Noodle Soup — 19
- Vegetable Soup Recipe — 20
- Minestrone Soup — 21
- Homemade French Onion Soup — 22
- Mac and Cheese Soup — 23
- Cheesy Potato Soup — 24
- Ham Bone Soup (Slow Cooker) — 25
- Quick Cabbage Soup — 26

27 DESSERT
- Homemade Cinnamon Roll Recipe — 28
- Peanut Butter Cake — 29
- Strawberry Pretzel Salad — 30
- Toll House Cookie Recipe — 31
- Homemade Brownies — 32
- Easy Red Velvet Cheesecake — 33
- No Churn Grape Ice Cream — 34
- Candied Pecans — 35
- Spritz Cookies — 36
- Chocolate Peppermint Cookies — 37

38 SLOW COOK
- CrockPot Spinach
- Crock Pot Pork Ch... — 40
- Ham and Bean Soup (Crock Pot Version) — 41
- Crock Pot Mac and Cheese — 42
- Crockpot Meatballs — 43
- Easy Crock Pot Chili Recipe — 44
- Crockpot Swiss Steak — 45
- Crock Pot Sausage Pasta — 46
- Crockpot Split Pea Soup — 47
- CrockPot Lasagna — 48

49 AIR FRYER
- Air Fryer Chicken Legs — 50
- Air Fryer Potato and Sausage — 51
- Air Fryer Spaghetti Squash — 52
- Air Fryer Stuffed Chicken Breasts — 53
- Lemon Pepper Wings — 54
- Air Fryer Roasted Garlic — 55
- Air Fryer Chicken Breasts — 56
- Air Fryer Pork Tenderloin — 57
- Bacon Wrapped Green Bean Bundles — 58
- Air Fryer Bacon Wrapped Brussels Sprouts — 59

60 BEVERAGE
- Copycat Baileys Recipe(Homemade Irish Cream) — 61
- Easy Mulled Wine Recipe — 61
- Bahama Mama &Green Kiwi Smoothie — 62
- Easy Red Sangria &Tequila Sunrise — 63
- Hot Chocolate Bombs — 64
- Copycat Shamrock Shake Recipe — 65
- Snickerdoodle Cocktail (with RumChata) — 65
- Champagne Punch &Kale Smoothie — 66
- Blueberry Smoothie — 67
- Fresh Homemade Limeade — 67
- Whipped Coffee (Dalgona) — 68
- Aperol Spritz — 68
- Dark and Stormy Cocktail — 69
- Classic Bloody Mary — 69
- Kir Royale Cocktail — 70
- Classic Martini Recipe — 70

TABLE OF CONTENTS

71 SALAD

- Easy Kale Salad with Fresh Lemon Dressing — 72, 73
- The Best Coleslaw Recipe — 74
- Chickpea Salad — 75
- Creamy Cranberry Salad — 76
- Old Fashioned Three Bean Salad — 77
- Brussels Sprout Salad — 78
- Avocado Corn Salad — 79
- Easy Arugula Salad — 80
- Easy Taco Salad — 81

82 INSTANT POT

- Instant Pot Minestrone Soup — 83
- Instant Pot Corned Beef — 84
- Instant Pot Spaghetti — 85
- Instant Pot Pot Roast — 86
- Instant Pot Lentil Soup — 87
- Instant Pot Mushroom Risotto — 88
- Instant Pot Turkey Breast — 89
- Instant Pot Egg Bites — 90
- Instant Pot Risotto — 91
- Instant Pot Cheesecake — 92
- Instant Pot Ribs — 93

94 DIP & DRESSING

- Baked Taco Ground Beef Dip — 95
- Easy Buffalo Chicken Dip (with canned chicken) — 96
- Easy Cheesy Pizza Dip — 97
- Easy Cheese Dip — 98
- Buffalo Ranch Chicken Dip — 99
- Quick & Easy Chocolate Hummus — 100
- Fluffy Pumpkin Dip — 101
- Mississippi Sin Dip — 102
- Easy Spinach Dip — 103
- Hot S'Mores Dip — 104

THE WEIGHT LOSS PROGRAM

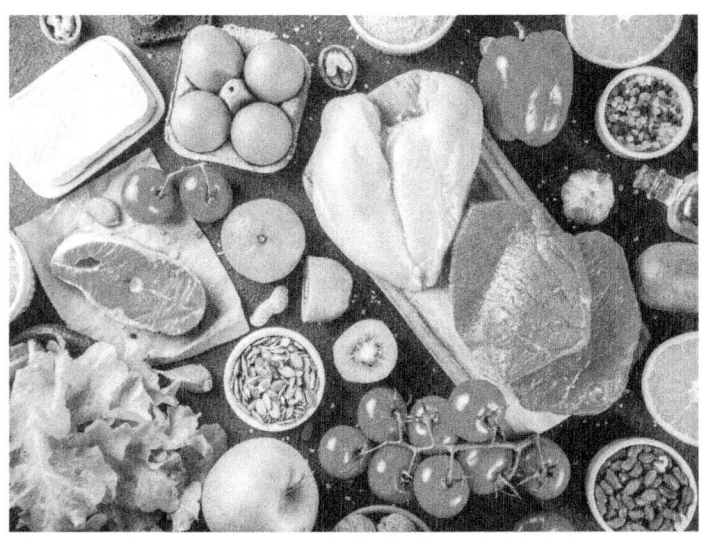

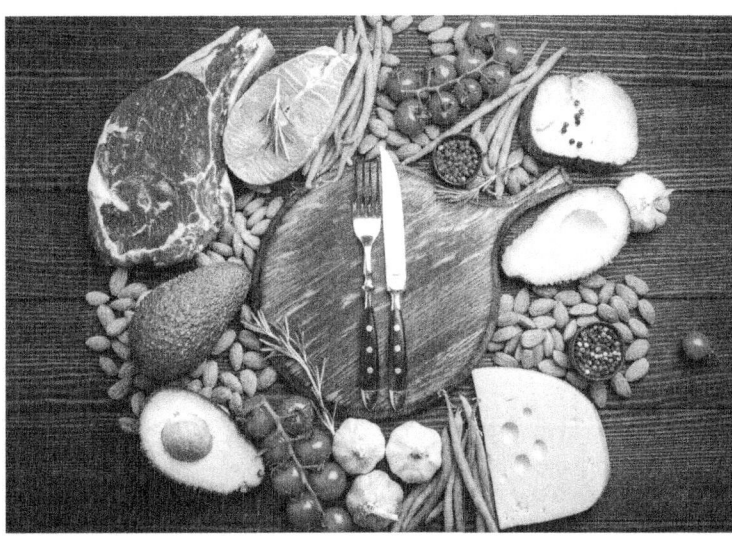

WHAT IS Weight Loss Program?

While losing weight isn't only about what you eat, Weight Loss Program realizes the critical role it plays in your success and overall good health. That's why our philosophy is to offer great-tasting, easy recipes that are nutritious as well as delicious. We create most of our recipes with the healthy and filling foods we love: lots of fresh fruits and vegetables, most of which have 0 Zero Point value, and satisfying lean proteins, which are low in Zero Point. We also try to ensure that our recipes fall within the recommendations of the U.S. Programary Guidelines for Americans so that they support a Program that promotes health and reduces the risk for disease. If you have special Programary needs, consult with your health-care professional for advice on a Program that is best for you, then adapt these recipes to meet your specific nutritional needs.

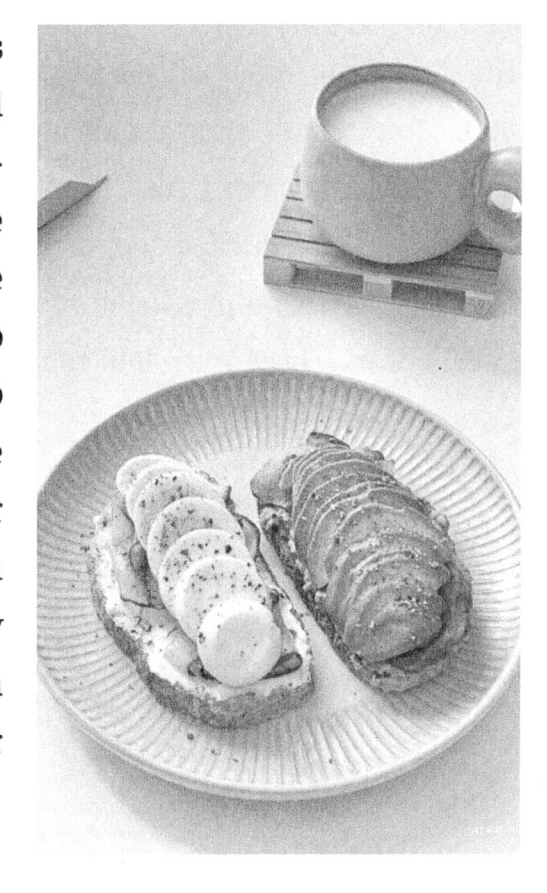

How does WW work?

Weight Loss Program uses a simplified calorie-counting system that is personalized based on your age, weight, height, and sex to help you lose weight in a healthy way. You track everything you eat and drink, as well as your workouts, on the app or website. Depending on your goal, you're allotted a specific number of what Weight Loss Program calls "Zero Point " each day. Every food and drink has a corresponding Zero Point value, with the healthiest foods being freebies with no Point at all—it's basically calorie counting with way less complicated math. Saturated fat and sugar drive the Zero Point value up, while protein drives it down. The aim is to guide you toward making better choices and, with practice, to make those choices habitual. In theory, if you consume the equivalent of your daily Zero Point (or below that number), you should lose weight, which you also record once a week on the Weight Loss Program platform.

Zero Point for the recipes in this book are calculated without counting any fruits and most vegetables, but the nutrition information does include the nutrient content from fruits and vegetables. This means you may get a different Zero Point value if you calculate the Zero Point based on the nutrition. To allow for your "free" fruits and veggies, use the Zero Point assigned to the recipes. Also, please note, when fruits and veggies are liquefied or pureed (as in a smoothie), their nutrient content is incorporated into the recipe calculations. These nutrients can increase the Zero Point.

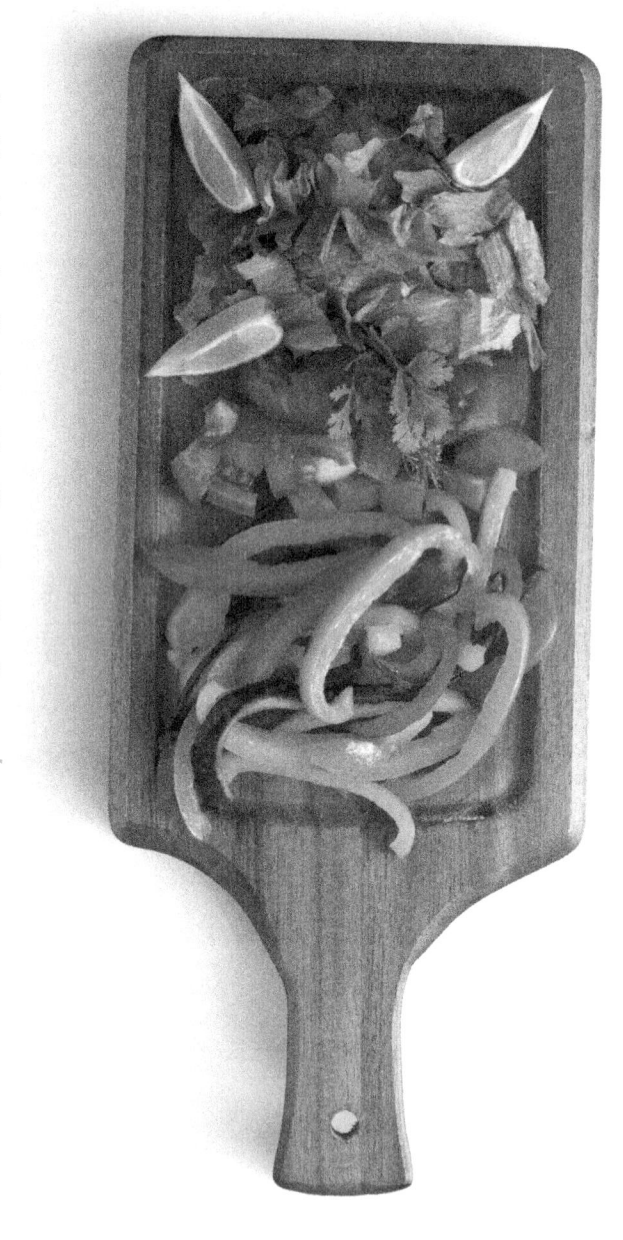

Will Weight Loss Program help you lose weight?

Most studies suggest Weight Loss Program is effective for Weight Loss Program, but may not be much more so than other similar Programs. Here's what several key studies had to say about Weight Loss Program:

- A study published in the May 2017 issue of Lancet of more than 1,200 overweight or obese patients in British primary care practices found that assigning participants to a WW for at least 12 weeks was more effective than providing brief advice and self-help materials for Weight Loss Program. A year-long program resulted in even more Weight Loss Program and was cost-effective, concluded the study supported by the U.K. National Prevention Research Initiative and Weight Loss Program International.

- A November 2014 review in Circulation: Cardiovascular Quality and Outcomes looked at the results of previous studies comparing Atkins, South Beach, Weight Loss Program and Zone Programs. It found that all but South Beach were equally effective at achieving sustained Weight Loss Program for more than a year. Weight Loss Program did have one advantage, though: In studies that compared it with usual care, rather than with other Programs, it was the only Program that "consistently demonstrated greater efficacy at reducing weight at 12 months," the researchers wrote.

- That finding supports a 2011 study in the Lancet showing that Weight Loss Program is more effective than standard weight-loss guidance. Researchers tracked 772 overweight and moderately obese people who either followed Weight Loss Program or got weight-loss guidance from their primary care doctors. After a year, those in the Weight Loss Program group had dropped 15 pounds compared with 7 pounds for the doctor-advised group. What's more, 61 percent of the Weight Loss Program participants stuck with the program for the full 12 months the study lasted, compared with 54 percent for the standard-care group. The program's success is likely explained by its regular weigh-ins and group meetings, which hold Programers accountable while offering support and motivation. Weight Loss Program funded the study, but an independent research team was responsible for all data collection and analysis.

- A 2013 study in the American Journal of Medicine also suggests Weight Loss Program has major benefits over standard "self-help" approaches. In it, researchers found overweight and obese participants assigned to Weight Loss Program were nearly nine times more likely to lose 10 percent of their weight than participants who were only provided with printed materials and publicly accessible websites and tools for Weight Loss Program. The more Weight Loss Program participants used the program's various tools – including meetings, a mobile phone app and online tools – the more weight they lost.

Shopping Guide

If you want to eat better and lose weight it's important to have healthy food on hand. Here's a great basic grocery shopping guide from Weight Loss Program to help get you started.

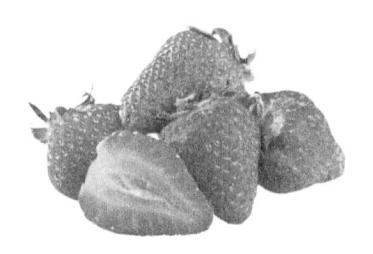

Produce

- Fresh fruit
- Bottled minced garlic
- Fresh lemons and limes to squeeze for juice
- Fresh vegetables (broccoli, celery, carrots, peppers, potatoes, green beans, squash, etc.)
- Fresh herbs (I like to grow my own in little pots on the windowsill - much cheaper)
- Packaged lettuce, coleslaw mix, spinach, etc.
- Pre-cut fresh vegetables for soups, stir-fries, snacks, dips, etc.

Bread

- Reduced-calorie bread or hamburger buns
- Thin sandwich bread or light English muffins
- Whole-wheat or corn tortillas

Deli

- Roasted whole chicken
- Lean reduced sodium deli meats

Grains/Pasta

- Whole-grain pasta (quinoa, brown rice, whole wheat, etc) or regular pasta
- Brown rice or white rice
- Bulgur, quinoa, barley, farro, etc
- Dry lentils (I like the precooked lentils at Trader Joes too)

Meat/Poultry/Fish (fresh and/or frozen without added sauce)

- Skinless chicken or turkey breast
- Ground turkey or chicken breast or 93% lean ground beef
- Lean center cut loin pork chops or pork tenderloin
- Canadian bacon
- Lean flank, strip, or sirloin steak, lean beef roasts; loin; or round cuts
- Tuna, wild salmon, flounder, scrod, cod, tilapia, haddock, halibut, etc.
- Shrimp, lobster, or scallops

Dairy

- Fat-free or low fat milk
- Regular soy milk (plain)
- Eggs or egg substitute
- Fat-free or low-fat cheese (shredded, slices, string, cottage, ricotta, etc)
- Fat-free or low-fat cream cheese
- Fat-free plain Greek yogurt
- Silken or firm regular or light tofu

Cereal

- Hot: Plain oatmeal, cream of wheat, multigrain or 100% bran
- Cold: Unsweetened shredded wheat, 100% whole-grain, or 100% bran

Canned Foods/Staples

- Tomato sauce or jarred marinara sauce
- Diced tomatoes with no added sugar
- Fat-free salsa
- Beans (black, pinto, white, etc) or chickpeas
- Canned vegetables (without added salt)
- Chopped chilies
- Canned artichoke hearts
- Fat-free low sodium broth
- Reduced-sodium light broth or tomato-based soups
- Canned unsweetened fruit (in water or juice)
- Pureed pumpkin for baking
- Tuna or salmon in water
- Peanut butter (no added sugar)
- Sugar-free jelly or jam (I buy "all fruit" spreads)

Dairy

- Light microwave (affiliate link) or air-popped popcorn
- Baked tortilla chips
- 100-calorie nut packs

Frozen

- Frozen vegetables (without added sauce or salt)
- Frozen unsweetened fruit
- Veggie burgers (with 2 g fat or less)
- Vegetarian ground "meat"
- Unsweetened fruit bars or ice pops

Seasonings & Condiments

- Cooking spray, oil, vinegar
- Salt and pepper
- Dried herbs and spices, seasoning mixes, and dry rubs
- Fat-free or low-fat salad dressing
- Fat-Free mayonnaise (I use low fat)
- Hot sauce
- Mustard
- Ketchup
- Fat free salsa
- Reduced sodium soy sauce
- Reduced sodium steak sauce
- Reduced-sodium teriyaki sauce

Chapter 1:
Breakfast

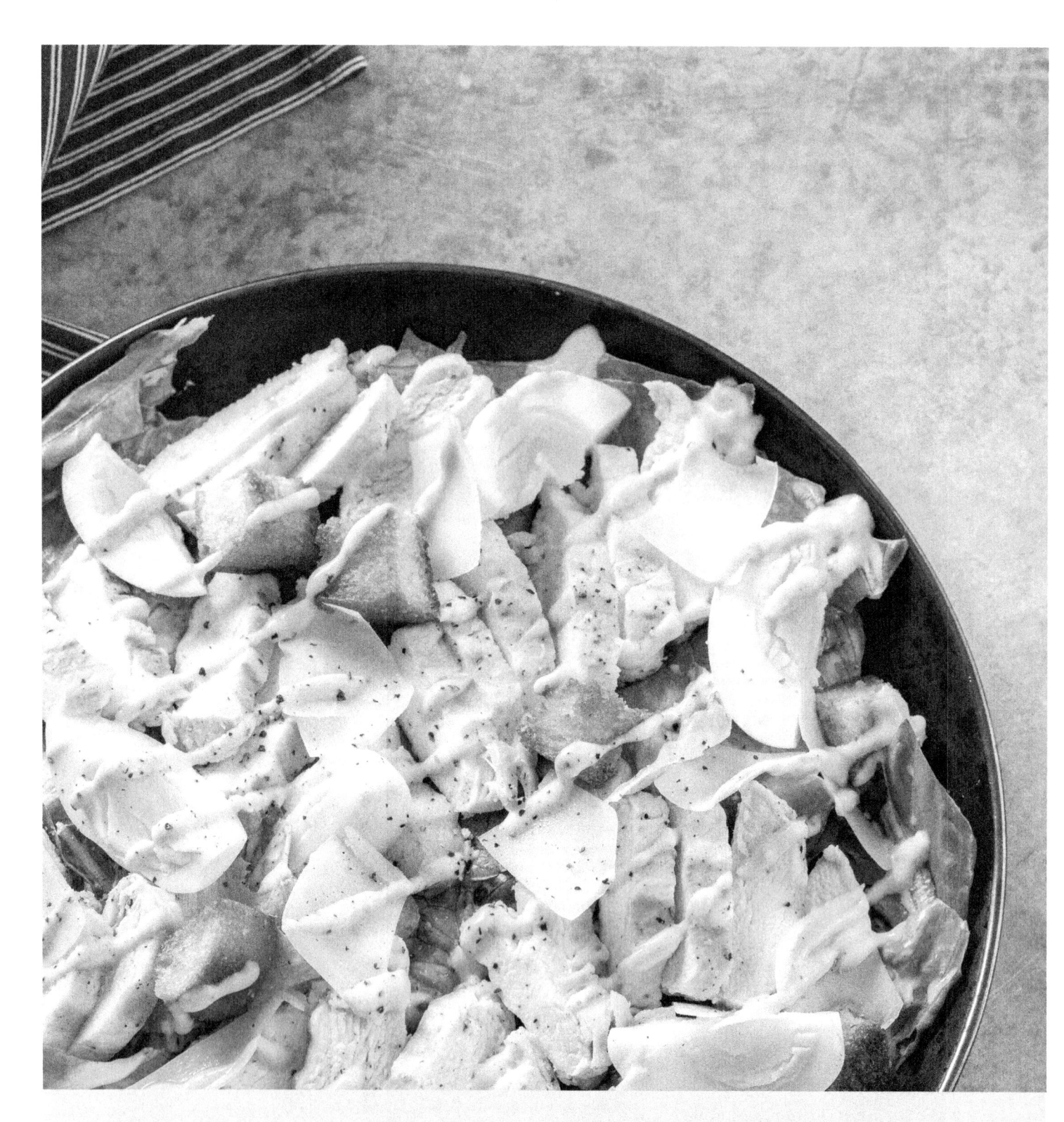

Blueberry French Toast Casserole

PREP TIME: 20 minutes **Serves:** 12
COOK TIME: 1 hour
CHILL TIME: 8 hours
TOTAL TIME: 9 hours 20 minutes

13

This French Toast Casserole is made with bread in an easy custard mixture, tossed with blueberries and a sweet cream cheese mixture, then topped with a sweet streusel topping!

Casserole
- 12 slices bread cut into 1-inch cubes
- 8 ounces cream cheese softened
- ¼ cup sugar
- 1 tablespoon lemon juice
- 1 ½ cups blueberries divided, fresh or frozen
- 12 eggs
- 2 cups milk
- ⅓ cup maple syrup
- 1 teaspoon lemon zest

Topping
- ½ cup oats
- ¼ cup butter softened
- ¼ cup flour
- 3 tablespoons brown sugar
- 3 tablespoons white sugar
- 1 teaspoon cinnamon

1. Leave your bread out for a few hours or place it on a tray at 350°F for about 8 minutes to slightly dry it out.
2. In a medium bowl, combine cream cheese, sugar and lemon juice until fluffy.
3. Grease a 9x13 inch baking dish. Layer half of the bread cubes in the pan. Top with cream cheese mixture & half the blueberries. Top with remaining bread and blueberries.
4. In a bowl, stir together the eggs, milk, syrup, and lemon zest until well mixed. Pour over the bread cubes, cover with foil, and refrigerate overnight.
5. Remove the casserole from the fridge about 45-60 minutes before baking. Preheat the oven to 350°F.
6. Mix topping ingredients together in a small bowl. Sprinkle over casserole just before baking.
7. Bake uncovered 45-55 minutes or until a knife inserted in the center comes out clean and is hot.

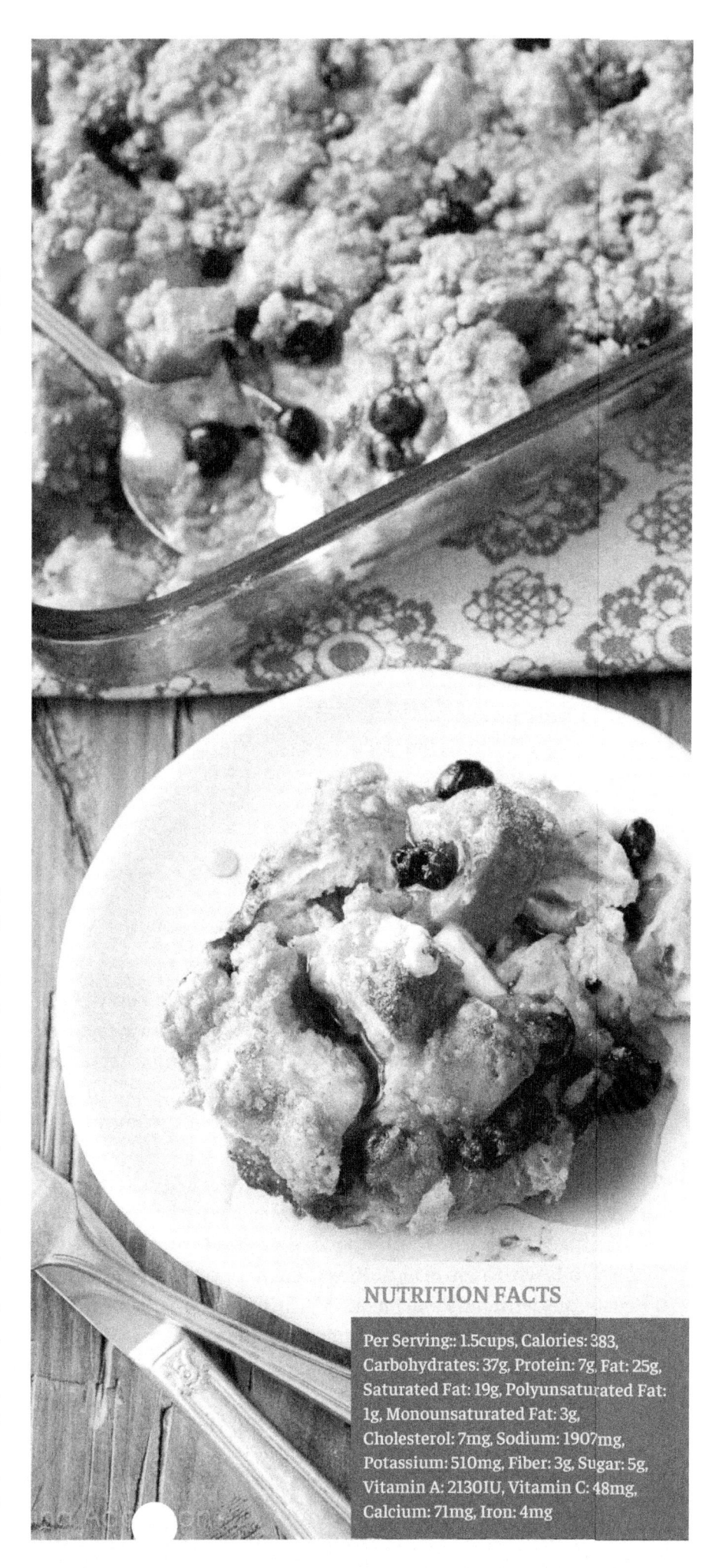

NUTRITION FACTS

Per Serving:: 1.5cups, Calories: 383, Carbohydrates: 37g, Protein: 7g, Fat: 25g, Saturated Fat: 19g, Polyunsaturated Fat: 1g, Monounsaturated Fat: 3g, Cholesterol: 7mg, Sodium: 1907mg, Potassium: 510mg, Fiber: 3g, Sugar: 5g, Vitamin A: 2130IU, Vitamin C: 48mg, Calcium: 71mg, Iron: 4mg

Homemade Cinnamon Roll Recipe

PREP TIME: 20 minutes Serves: 15
COOK TIME: 2 hours 30 minutes
TOTAL TIME: 2 hours 50 minutes

24

This recipe makes soft rolls with sticky-sweet cinnamon filling on the inside, and dripping with cream cheese icing on the outside!

- ¼ cup warm water
- 1 package active dry yeast or 2 ¼ teaspoons
- ¾ cup whole milk
- ⅓ cup butter
- ⅓ cup granulated sugar plus 1 teaspoon
- ½ teaspoon salt
- 3 ¾ to 4 ¼ cups all purpose flour divided
- 2 eggs room temperature

Filling
- ½ cup butter softened
- 1 cup brown sugar packed
- 2 tablespoons ground cinnamon

Frosting
- 1 ½ cups powdered sugar or as needed
- 4 ounces cream cheese softened
- ¼ cup unsalted butter softened
- ½ teaspoon vanilla extract
- ⅛ teaspoon salt

1. Grease a 9x13 pan or baking dish.
2. Combine water, yeast, and 1 teaspoon sugar in a small bowl. Let sit 10 minutes or until foamy.
3. Combine milk, butter, remaining sugar, and salt in a saucepan and heat to 120-130°F.
4. Place 2 cups flour in a stand mixer. Add eggs, milk mixture, and yeast mixture. Mix until combined.
5. Using a dough hook, add flour, ½ cup at a time, to form a soft dough that pulls away from the side of the bowl. Remove dough from the bowl and knead on a lightly floured surface until dough is smooth and elastic (approx. 8 mins).
6. Place in a greased bowl in a warm spot and cover with a towel for 1 hour or until doubled in size.
7. Roll dough into a 15" x 12" rectangle, spread butter on the dough and top with brown sugar and cinnamon.
8. Roll dough starting on the long side. Slice into 15 pieces. Place in prepared pan.
9. Cover rolls with a towel and allow them to rise 30-45 minutes. Preheat oven to 375°F.
10. Brush rolls with milk and bake 20-25 minutes.
11. While the rolls are baking, combine powdered sugar, cream cheese, butter, vanilla extract, and salt with a mixer until fluffy.

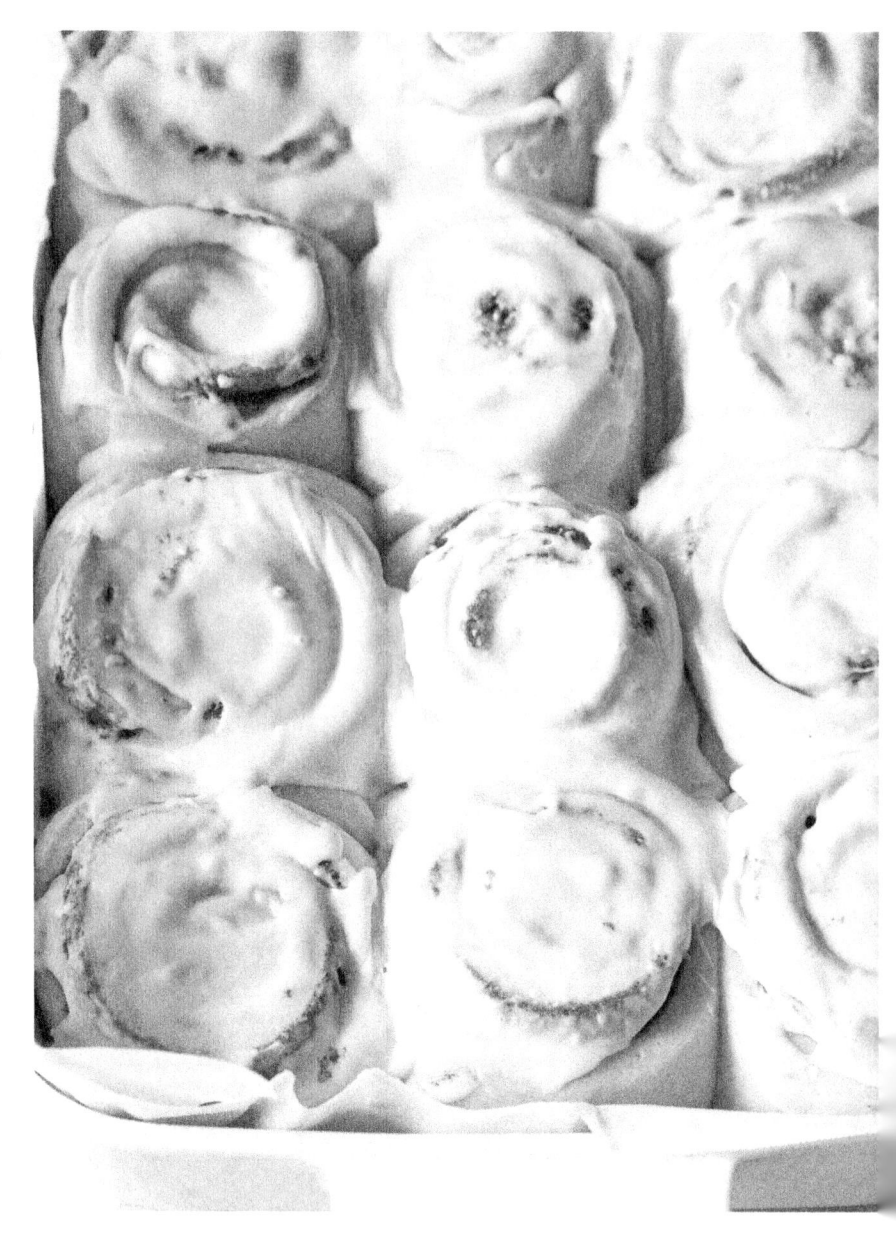

NUTRITION FACTS

Calories: 406, Carbohydrates: 59g, Protein: 6g, Fat: 17g, Saturated Fat: 10g, Cholesterol: 66mg, Sodium: 257mg, Potassium: 103mg, Fiber: 2g, Sugar: 30g, Vitamin A: 566IU, Calcium: 58mg, Iron: 2mg

Tater Tot Breakfast Casserole

PREP TIME: 15 minutes Serves: 8
COOK TIME: 1 hour 15 minutes
CHILL TIME: 8 hours
TOTAL TIME: 9 hours 30 minutes

22

Loaded with fresh peppers, bacon, & cheese, this Tater Tot Breakfast Casserole is perfect for serving to a crowd!

- 20 ounces tater tots
- 1 pound bacon or 1 pound sausage *see note
- 1 onion diced
- 1 red bell pepper diced
- 1 green bell pepper diced
- 6 eggs
- ⅔ cup milk
- ½ teaspoon garlic powder
- ¼ teaspoon kosher salt
- ¼ teaspoon black pepper
- 3 cups Mexican blend shredded cheese or shredded cheddar cheese, divided

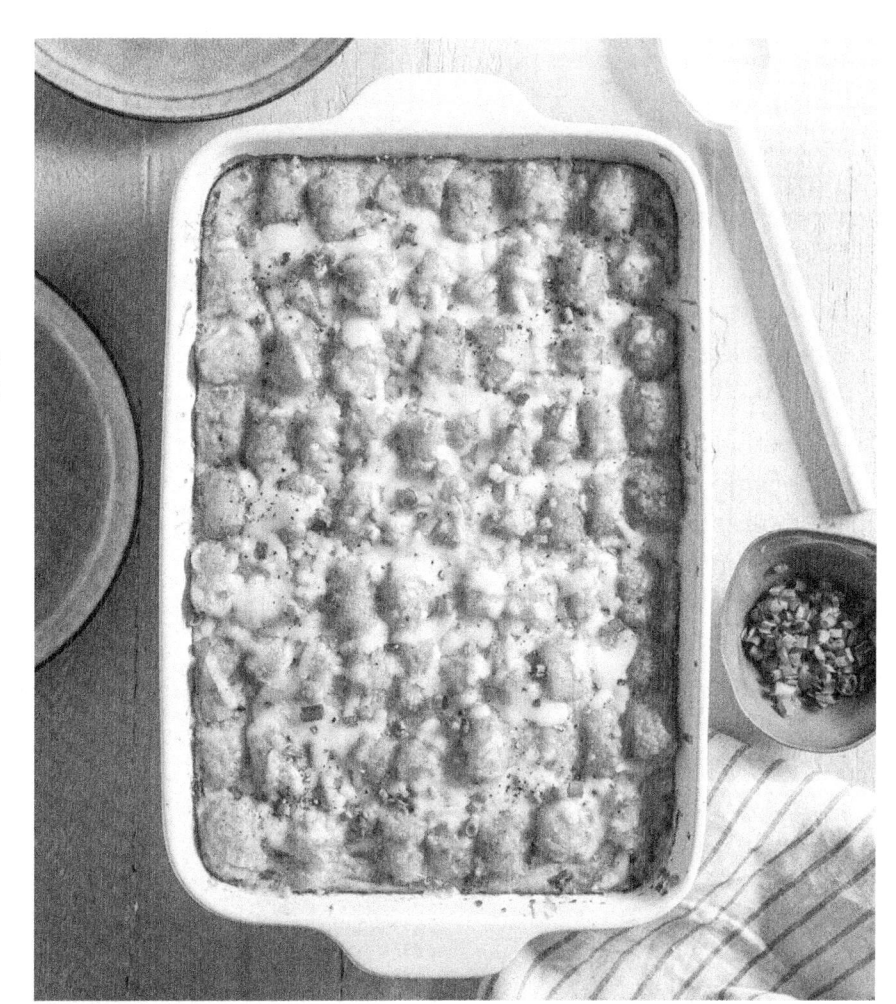

1. Spread the tater tots in a single layer in a greased 9x13 pan. Sprinkle 1 cup of cheese over the tots.
2. Chop the bacon into 1" pieces and cook in a medium skillet until crisp. Remove the bacon to a paper towel-lined plate, leaving 2 tablespoons of bacon fat in the pan.
3. Add onion to the pan and cook over medium heat until softened. Add the bell peppers and stir to combine. Sprinkle over the tater tots along with ⅔ of the bacon.
4. Whisk eggs, milk, garlic powder, salt, & pepper in a bowl. Pour over the tater tots.
5. Cover tightly with foil and refrigerate overnight.
6. Preheat the oven to 350°F. Bake the covered casserole for 40 minutes. Remove the cover, top with remaining cheese and bacon. Turn the oven up to 425°F and bake an additional 15-20 minutes or until set and cheese is browned.

Recipe Notes
1. Cheese can be replaced with 2 cups pepper jack and 1 cup cheddar cheese.
2. If using sausage, cook the onion and sausage together. Drain any fat.

Time Saving Tips
1. Use precooked bacon or ham
2. Frozen onions and peppers can be used in place of fresh.
3. Pre-shredded cheese works in this recipe
4. Use frozen tater tots, no need to thaw first
5. Remove the casserole from the fridge up to an hour before baking.

NUTRITION FACTS

Calories: 572, Carbohydrates: 20g, Protein: 25g, Fat: 44g, Saturated Fat: 17g, Polyunsaturated Fat: 6g, Monounsaturated Fat: 17g, Trans Fat: 1g, Cholesterol: 242mg, Sodium: 1056mg, Potassium: 469mg, Fiber: 2g, Sugar: 3g, Vitamin A: 1098IU, Vitamin C: 36mg, Calcium: 342mg, Iron: 2mg

Sausage Breakfast Casserole

PREP TIME: 20 minutes
COOK TIME: 1 hour 25 minutes
TOTAL TIME: 1 hour 45 minutes
Serves: 10

18

Sausage Breakfast Casserole is loaded with eggs, sausage, and hashbrowns for a hearty breakfast that's perfect for a crowd!

- 1 pound breakfast sausages or bulk sausage
- 1 large onion diced
- 20 ounces diced hash browns thawed
- 1 red bell pepper diced
- 4 ounces mild green chiles drained
- 1 cup pepper jack cheese shredded, divided
- 1 cup cheddar cheese shredded, divided

Egg Mixture

- 8 eggs
- 1 ⅓ cups milk
- ½ teaspoon cumin
- ½ teaspoon garlic powder
- salt & pepper to taste

1. Preheat oven to 350°F (if baking immediately). Grease a 9x13 pan or a 3qt casserole dish.
2. If using breakfast sausage links, cut the breakfast sausages into 4 pieces about ½-inch long.
3. Place sausages in a large skillet and cook over medium-high heat until are browned, about 7-8 minutes. Add onion to the pan and cook until the sausages are cooked through and the onion is softened, about 3 minutes more. Drain any fat and set aside to cool.
4. Place the sausage mixture, thawed hash browns, bell pepper, green chiles, and half of each of the cheeses in the prepared pan. Stir to combine.
5. Whisk the egg mixture in a large bowl until smooth. Pour over the hashbrowns.
6. Cover and refrigerate overnight* if desired or bake immediately.
7. Bake covered for 40 minutes. Uncover, top with remaining 1 cup of cheese, and bake an additional 30-35 minutes or until cooked through.

Recipe Notes

1. If casserole is refrigerated overnight, remove it from the fridge 30 minutes before baking. It may require an extra 10-15 minutes cooking time.
2. Frozen diced potatoes make this quick and easy. If you'd like to use your own fresh potatoes, peel and dice 1/2". Cook the diced potatoes (either boil, roast, or panfry) until tender. Shredded hashbrowns work too.
3. If adding other vegetables, be sure to pre-cook any that have a lot of water (like mushrooms).
4. Remove the casserole from the fridge while the oven preheats.
5. After baking, let the casserole rest for about 10-15 minutes before cutting into squares and serving.

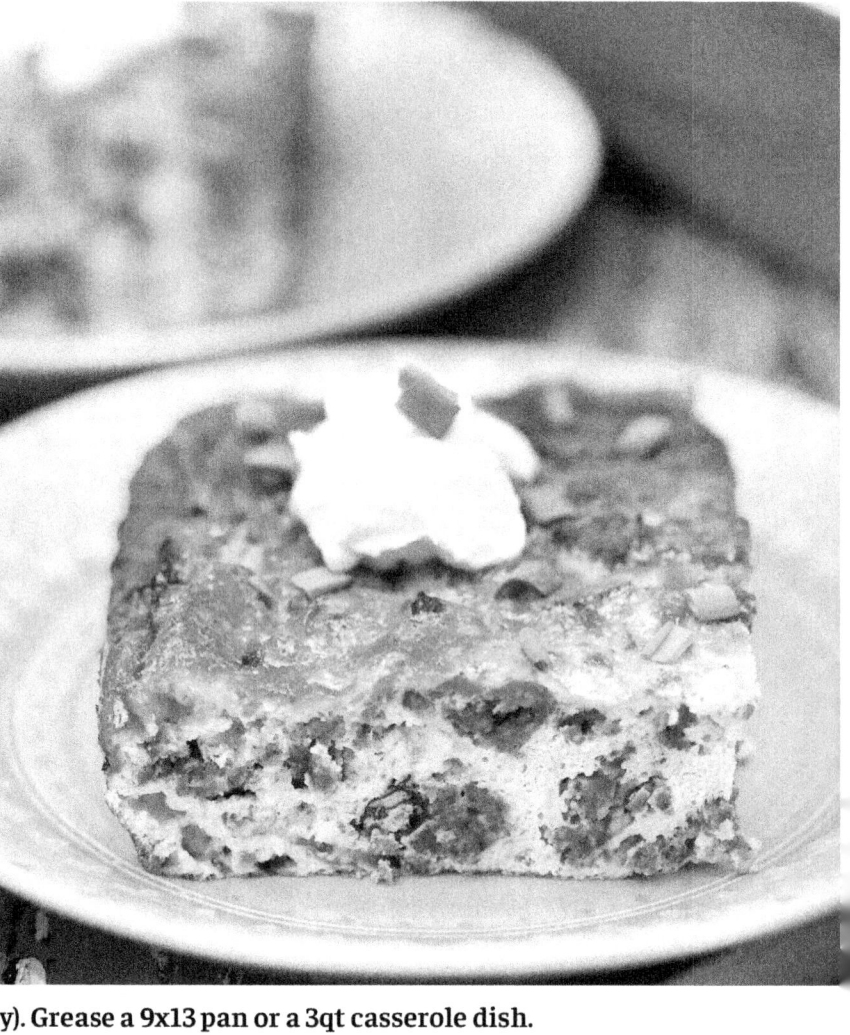

NUTRITION FACTS

Calories: 451, Carbohydrates: 25g, Protein: 20g, Fat: 30g, Saturated Fat: 11g, Polyunsaturated Fat: 5g, Monounsaturated Fat: 12g, Trans Fat: 1g, Cholesterol: 187mg, Sodium: 716mg, Potassium: 600mg, Fiber: 3g, Sugar: 4g, Vitamin A: 863IU, Vitamin C: 25mg, Calcium: 241mg, Iron: 2mg

Fluffy Homemade Waffle Recipe

PREP TIME: 15 minutes   Serves: 6
COOK TIME: 10 minutes
TOTAL TIME: 25 minutes

6

Nothing beats them for home-cooked comfort and making the kids or weekend guests feel special.

- 2 cups flour
- 1 tablespoon baking powder
- ½ teaspoon salt
- 2 tablespoons sugar
- 2 eggs divided
- 1 ⅔ cup milk
- ⅓ cup melted butter or oil

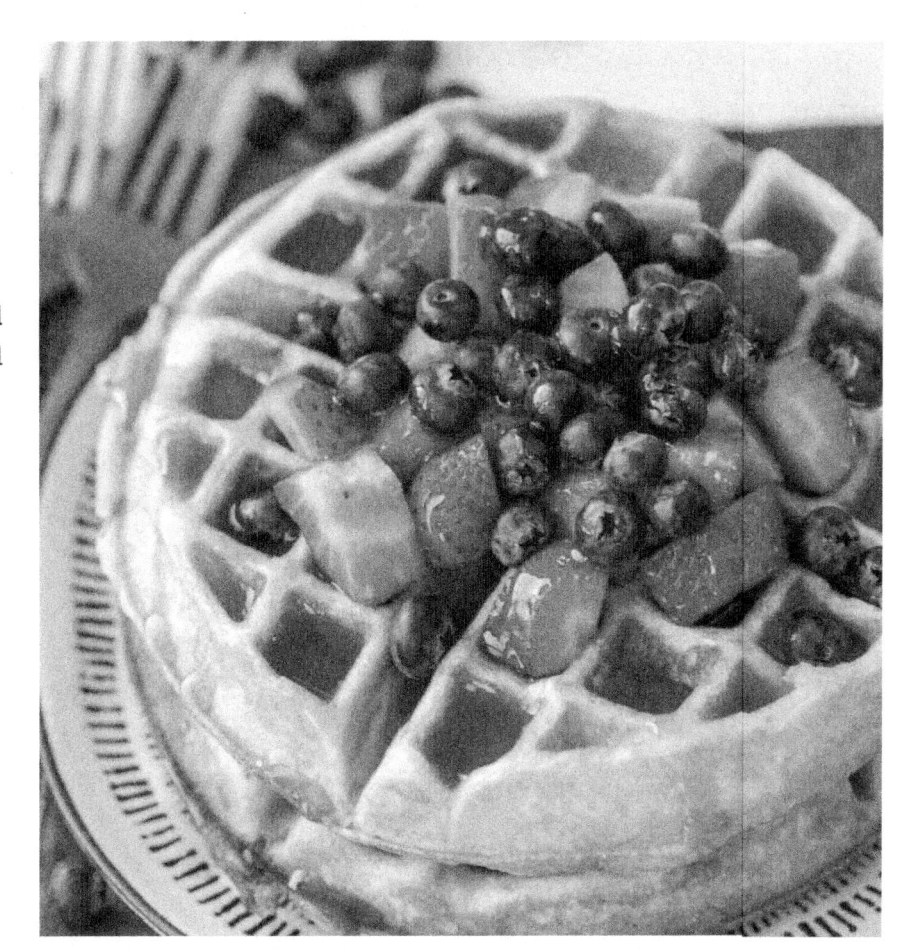

1. Preheat the waffle iron according to the manufacturer's directions.
2. Place flour, baking powder, sugar, and salt in a bowl. Whisk to combine.
3. In a small bowl, mix egg yolks, milk, and butter. Set aside.
4. In a separate bowl, beat egg whites with a mixer on medium high speed until stiff peaks form. *see note
5. Add egg yolk mixture to flour mixture and stir to combine. Fold in egg whites.
6. Drop by large spoonfuls onto greased waffle iron, close the lid and cook about 3-5 minutes.

Recipe Notes

1. Beating the egg whites and folding them in makes the fluffiest waffles. This recipe can be made without beating the egg whites as well. If you do not beat the egg whites, reduce milk to 1 1/2 cups, and add whole eggs to the butter mixture.
2. To Keep Warm if Making Batches
3. Preheat the oven to 225°F and place a baking pan in the oven. As the waffles are finished cooking, place them on the baking pan to stay warm while you make the remaining waffles.
4. Buttermilk Waffles
5. To make buttermilk waffles, reduce baking powder to 1 1/2 teaspoons and add 1/2 teaspoon baking soda. Replace milk with buttermilk.
6. Tips for the Best Waffles
7. Don't overmix the batter, it should be lumpy.
8. Preheat the waffle maker and lightly oil with vegetable oil. Do not use cooking spray.
9. Put enough batter in the iron so the waffle is almost full, it will run out to the edges a little bit.

NUTRITION FACTS

Calories: 308, Carbohydrates: 40g, Protein: 8g, Fat: 13g, Saturated Fat: 7g, Cholesterol: 85mg, Sodium: 336mg, Potassium: 365mg, Fiber: 1g, Sugar: 8g, Vitamin A: 523IU, Calcium: 186mg, Iron: 2mg

Chorizo Breakfast Hash

PREP TIME: 45 minutes   **Serves:** 6
COOK TIME: 15 minutes
TOTAL TIME: 1 hour

`16`

Start the day off right with this easy Chorizo Breakfast Hash! Spicy sausage and smoky bacon are cooked with creamy potatoes, then topped with scrambled egg and cheese.

- 2 pounds Yukon gold potatoes ½ inch pieces
- 1 pound chorizo sausage casing removed
- 4 strips bacon sliced
- 1 onion diced
- 4 cloves garlic minced
- 1 teaspoon coriander
- 1 teaspoon cumin
- ¾ teaspoon smoked paprika
- 6 eggs whisked
- 1 cup cheddar cheese shredded

1. Preheat the oven to 375°F.
2. Place the potatoes in a large pot with 6 cups of water, bring to a boil and cook for 6-8 minutes or until they are fork tender. Drain them and set aside.
3. While potatoes are cooking, heat a large skillet over medium heat. Cook the bacon until crisp. Remove and set aside.
4. Remove the casing from the chorizo and add it to the bacon fat along with the onion. Cook until no pink remains, about 8 minutes. Remove from the pan and set aside leaving the fat in the pan.
5. Turn the heat up to medium high and add the potatoes, seasonings, and garlic to the pan. Cook until browned without stirring too much so the potatoes can form a crust. Stir in the meat.
6. While potatoes are browning, lightly scramble the eggs in a small pan over medium heat. Eggs should be slightly undercooked and shiny. Place on top of the hash and sprinkle cheese on top.
7. Place in the oven and heat until cheese is melted and heat through, about 5 minutes.

Recipe Notes
1. This pork sausage can be either spicy or sweet, choose the flavor that you prefer. Be sure to remove the casing when preparing the sausage for this recipe. Bacon adds a smoky crisp to this recipe.
2. Potatoes can be replaced with leftover potatoes or a bag of frozen homestyle hash browns. If using frozen potatoes or leftovers, you can skip boiling the potatoes.
3. Optional Topping Ideas
4. corn tortillas, sour cream, diced tomatoes, green onions, jalapeno, shredded cabbage, guacamole, salsa, cheese, cilantro.

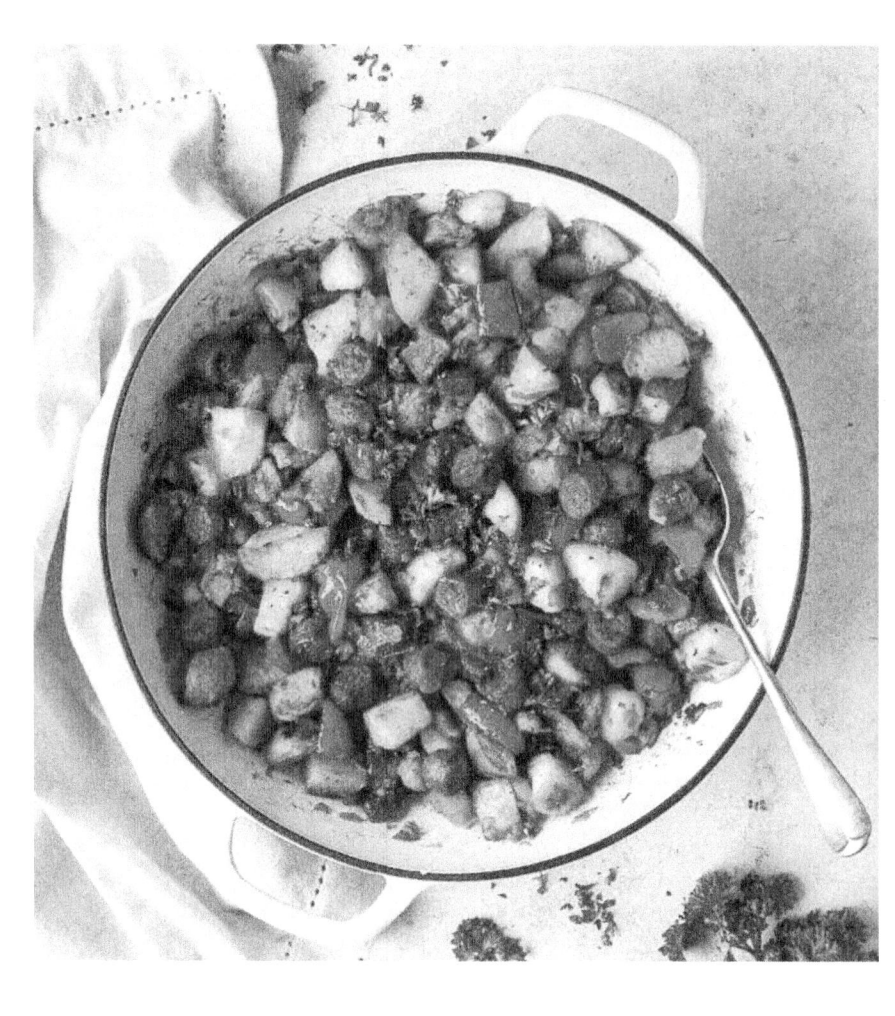

NUTRITION FACTS

Calories: 451, Carbohydrates: 30g, Protein: 22g, Fat: 26g, Saturated Fat: 13g, Polyunsaturated Fat: 2g, Monounsaturated Fat: 6g, Trans Fat: 1g, Cholesterol: 246mg, Sodium: 1400mg, Potassium: 792mg, Fiber: 4g, Sugar: 2g, Vitamin A: 945IU, Vitamin C: 46mg, Calcium: 206mg, Iron: 3mg

Homemade Shredded Hashbrowns

PREP TIME: 20 minutes
COOK TIME: 20 minutes
TOTAL TIME: 40 minutes
Serves: 9

`3`

Homemade Shredded Hashbrowns are pan-fried to a crispy golden brown perfection. So easy to make, they are the perfect addition to every brunch.

- 3 medium russet potatoes peeled
- 2 eggs
- 1 teaspoon garlic powder
- salt and pepper to taste
- 2 tablespoons vegetable oil

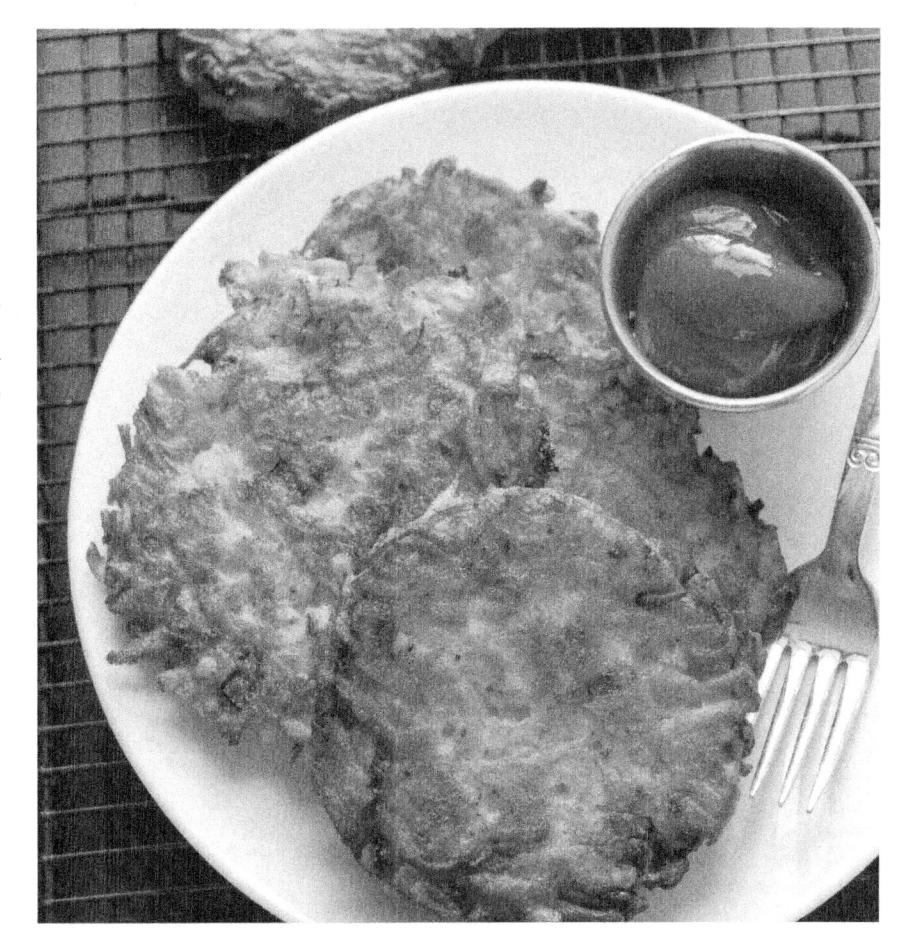

1. Preheat oven to 350°F.
2. Shred potatoes using the large side of a box grater.
3. Rinse potatoes in a strainer. Place in a large bowl of cold water and let sit for 5 minutes. Drain very well and squeeze potatoes dry.
4. Combine eggs, potatoes, and seasonings together in a medium bowl.
5. Heat vegetable oil over medium-high heat in a large skillet. Scoop ¼ cup mounds of potato mixture into the pan and flatten slightly with the back of a spoon.
6. Cook each side until golden brown, about 4-5 minutes per side. Place browned hashbrowns on a baking sheet and cook an additional 10-15 minutes or until tender.

Recipe Notes

1. Soak and squeeze well. Soaking the hashbrowns removes excess starch keeping the potatoes fluffy as they cook.
2. When squeezing the water out of the hashbrowns, place the potatoes in a tea towel and twist to squeeze out the water (rinse the kitchen towel well, potatoes can stain the towel).
3. An egg is optional but we find the potatoes hold together best this way.

NUTRITION FACTS

Serving: 1hashbrown patty, Calories: 99, Carbohydrates: 13g, Protein: 3g, Fat: 4g, Saturated Fat: 1g, Polyunsaturated Fat: 1g, Monounsaturated Fat: 3g, Trans Fat: 1g, Cholesterol: 36mg, Sodium: 18mg, Potassium: 314mg, Fiber: 1g, Sugar: 1g, Vitamin A: 54IU, Vitamin C: 4mg, Calcium: 15mg, Iron: 1mg

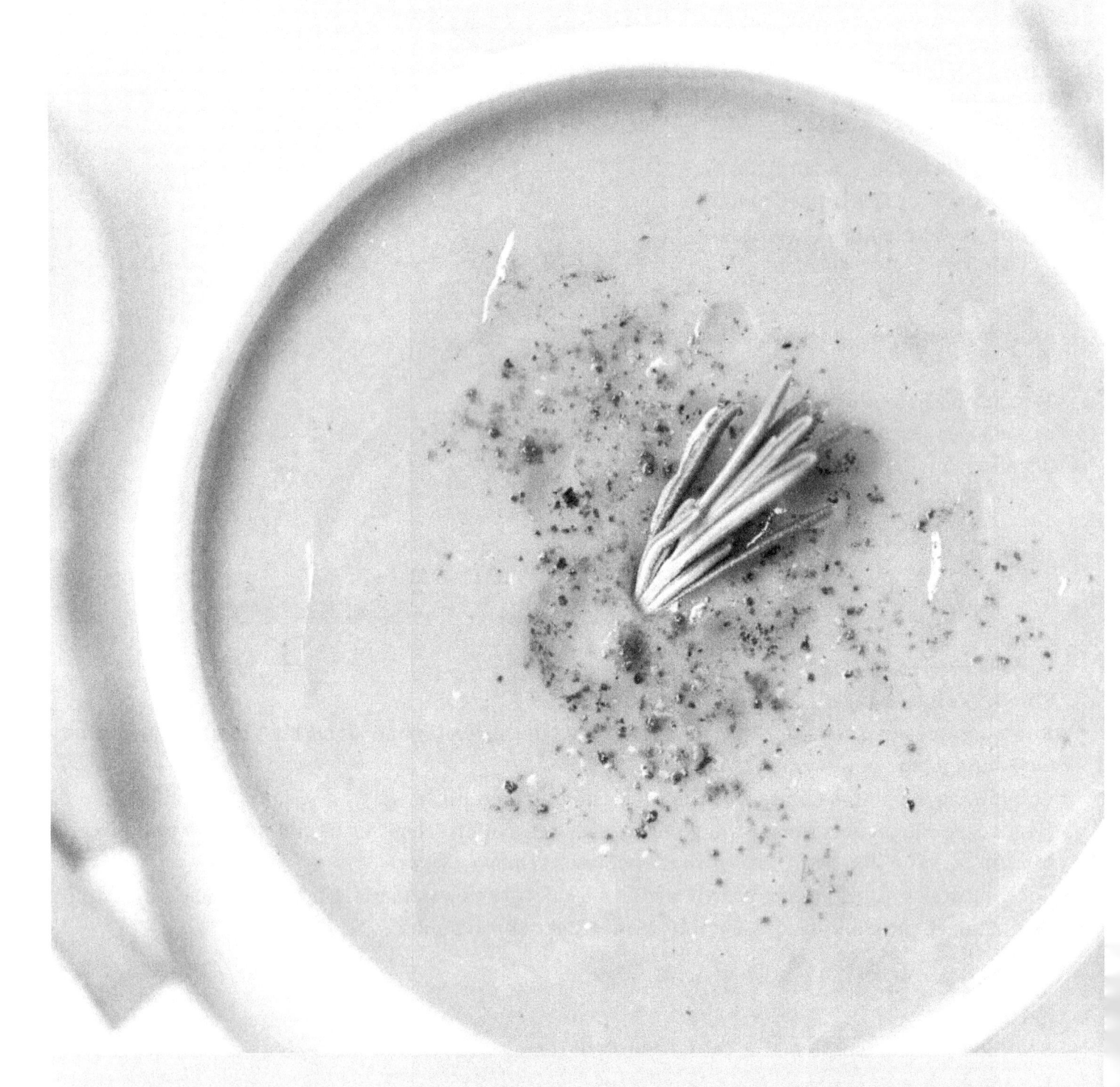

Chapter 2:
Soup

Coconut Curry Soup

PREP TIME: 20 minutes **Serves:** 4
COOK TIME: 30 minutes
TOTAL TIME: 50 minutes

Made with shrimp, veggies, Thai red curry paste, and coconut milk, this soup is bursting with Asian-inspired flavors!

- t2 teaspoons vegetable oil
- 1 lime divided use
- 1 medium onion sliced
- 2 tablespoons Thai red curry paste
- 1 ½ tablespoons minced fresh ginger
- 4 cloves garlic minced
- 4 cups chicken broth
- 14 ounces coconut milk do not use light or low fat
- 1 ½ tablespoons fish sauce
- ¾ cup mushrooms thinly sliced
- 1 red bell pepper thinly sliced
- 8 ounces uncooked peeled medium shrimp or 2 cups cooked chicken
- 4 ounces medium rice noodles cooked
- fresh herbs for serving, optional cilantro, Thai basil, fresh mint

1. Zest 1 teaspoon of lime zest and set aside. Juice half of the lime (about 1 tablespoon of juice) and reserve the rest for serving.
2. Heat vegetable oil in a large saucepan over medium heat. Add sliced onion to the pan and cook until it begins to soften, about 4 minutes.
3. Add curry paste, ginger, and garlic and stir until fragrant, about 2 minutes.
4. Stir in chicken broth, coconut milk, and fish sauce, scraping up any brown bits. Add mushrooms and lime zest, simmer 15 minutes.
5. Add bell pepper and rice noodles* (see note), simmer for 3 minutes more.
6. Stir in raw shrimp or cooked chicken, turn off the heat, and cover. Let rest 5-6 minutes or until shrimp is cooked through or chicken is heated through and the noodles have softened.
7. Stir in the juiced lime. Serve with fresh herbs and additional lime wedges.

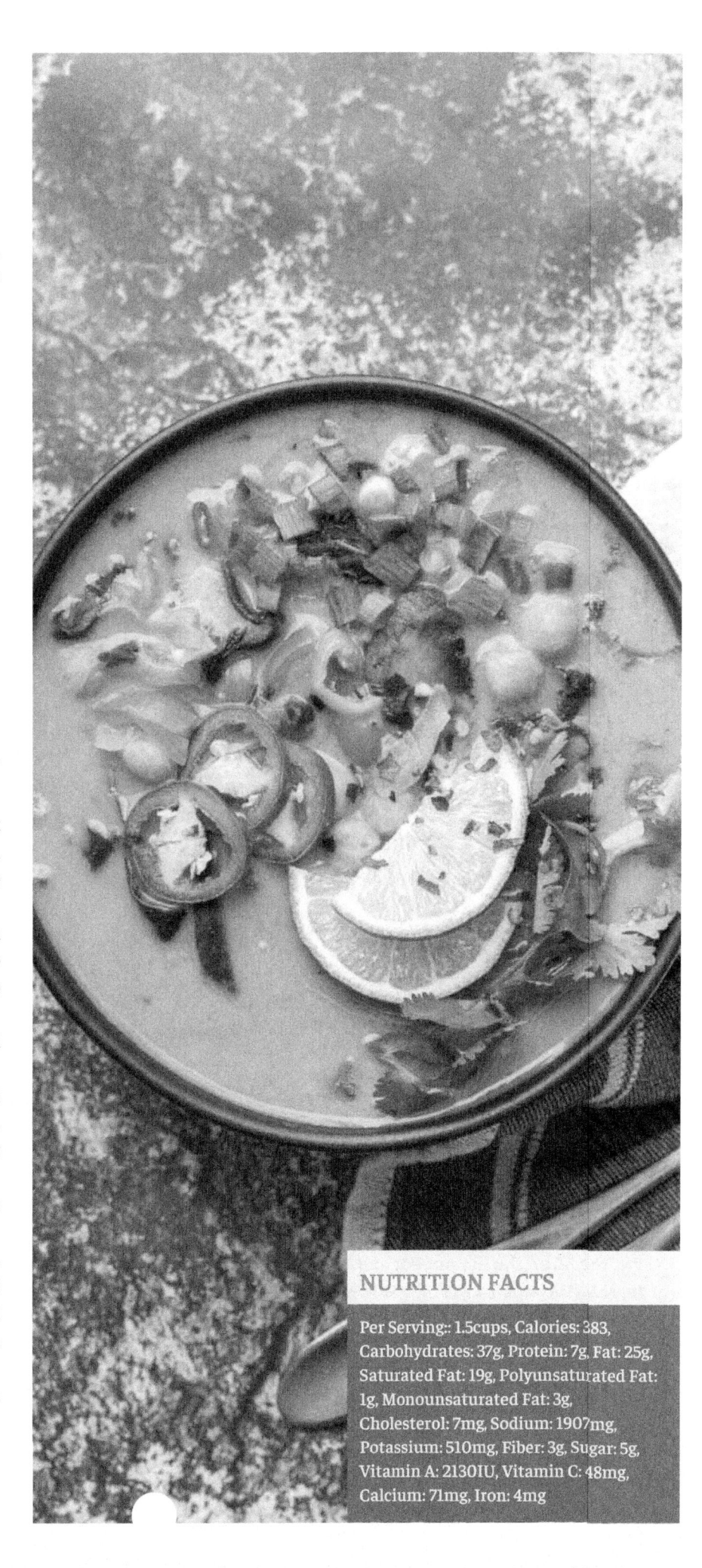

NUTRITION FACTS

Per Serving:: 1.5cups, Calories: 383, Carbohydrates: 37g, Protein: 7g, Fat: 25g, Saturated Fat: 19g, Polyunsaturated Fat: 1g, Monounsaturated Fat: 3g, Cholesterol: 7mg, Sodium: 1907mg, Potassium: 510mg, Fiber: 3g, Sugar: 5g, Vitamin A: 2130IU, Vitamin C: 48mg, Calcium: 71mg, Iron: 4mg

Minestrone Soup

PREP TIME: 20 minutes
COOK TIME: 20 minutes   Serves: 6
TOTAL TIME: 40 minutes

10

We love this easy Minestrone Soup loaded with healthy, colorful veggies and cooked in the Instant Pot!

- 1 tablespoon oil vegetable or olive
- 1 onion finely diced
- 3 large carrots chopped
- 2 ribs celery sliced
- 6 cups low sodium chicken broth
- 28 ounces canned diced tomatoes with juice
- 15.5 ounces canned red kidney beans drained and rinsed
- 15.5 ounces canned cannellini beans drained and rinsed
- 1 ½ cups mini shell pasta uncooked
- ½ zucchini sliced into ½" half moons
- 2 cloves garlic minced
- 1 ½ teaspoons salt
- 1 ½ teaspoons dried Italian seasoning
- 2 bay leaves
- ⅛ teaspoon black pepper
- 2 cups fresh spinach chopped
- fresh basil, parsley, and/or parmesan cheese for serving optional

1. Turn a 6 qt Instant Pot onto SAUTÉ.
2. Once heated, add oil, onion, carrots, and celery. Cook while stirring until the onions are slightly softened, about 3 minutes.
3. Add broth and use a spatula to scrape up any brown bits in the bottom of the Instant Pot.
4. Add remaining ingredients except for the spinach & basil if using.
5. Put the lid on the Instant Pot and set it to MANUAL (or PRESSURE COOK) on HIGH pressure for 4 minutes.
6. When the cooking time is done, quick release the pressure and open the lid. Stir in spinach and let rest 5-10 minutes.
7. Remove the bay leaves and discard.
8. Serve with shredded parmesan cheese and fresh basil or parsley if desired.

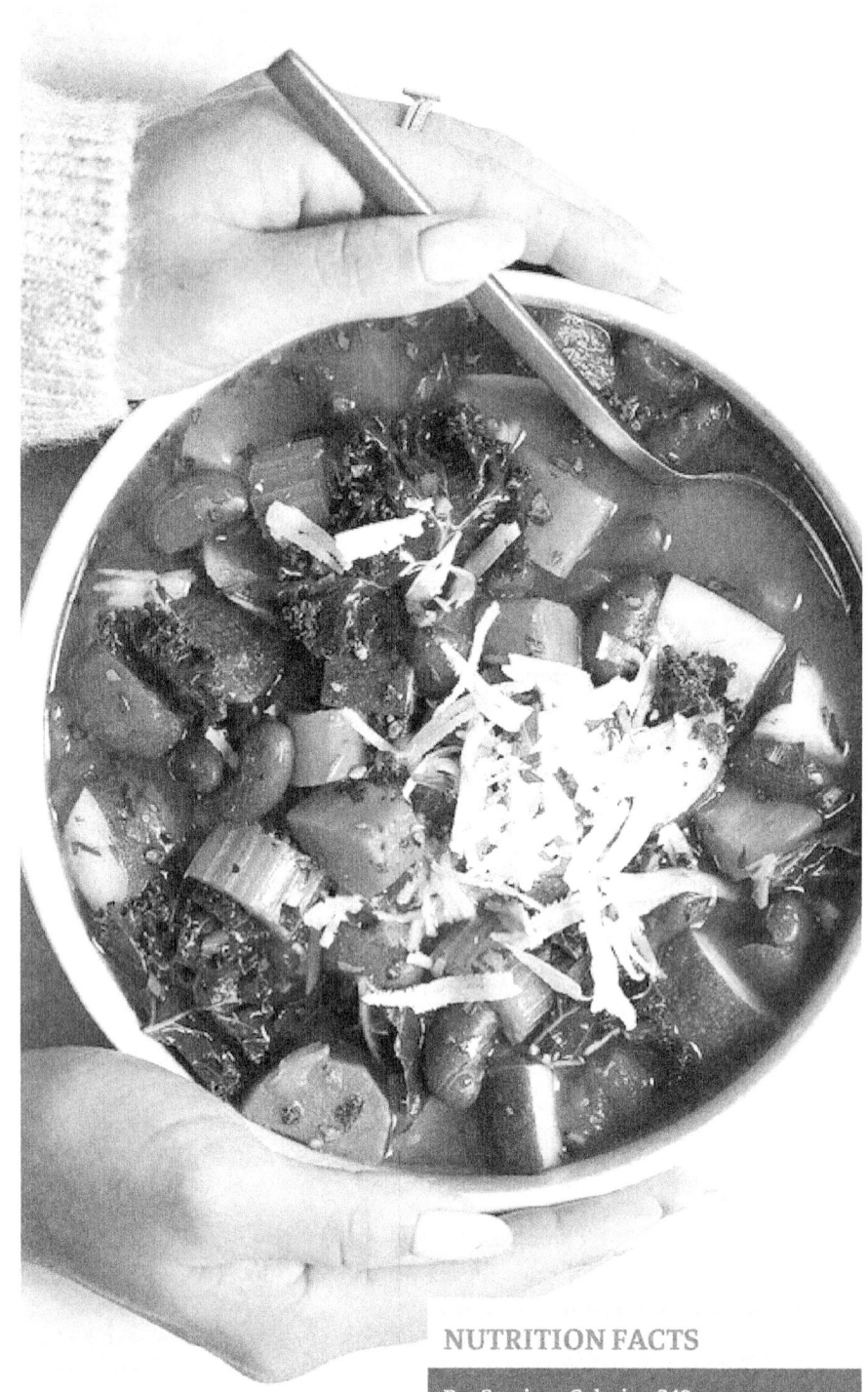

NUTRITION FACTS

Per Serving:: Calories: 349, Carbohydrates: 60g, Protein: 19g, Fat: 5g, Saturated Fat: 1g, Polyunsaturated Fat: 2g, Monounsaturated Fat: 2g, Trans Fat: 1g, Sodium: 1080mg, Potassium: 1317mg, Fiber: 12g, Sugar: 9g, Vitamin A: 7210IU, Vitamin C: 23mg, Calcium: 175mg, Iron: 6mg

Chicken Noodle Soup

PREP TIME: 20 minutes **Serves:** 6
COOK TIME: 15 minutes
TOTAL TIME: 2 hr 5 minutes

3

Heartwarming and hearty chicken noodle soup is perfect for chilly days!

- 8 cups chicken broth or chicken stock (*see note)
- 1 ½ cups carrots sliced
- 1 cup celery sliced
- 3-4 cups cooked chicken or chicken below
- 2 cups egg noodles measured dry
- salt & freshly ground black pepper to taste

Homemade Chicken Broth:
- 1 whole chicken 3-4 lbs
- 1 ½ onions divided
- 3 carrots include tops if you have them
- 2 stalks celery
- 4 sprigs fresh herbs rosemary, parsley, sage (or any combination)
- 2 bay leaves
- 1 tablespoon peppercorns
- 2 teaspoons salt
- 1 teaspoon poultry seasoning
- 10 cups water

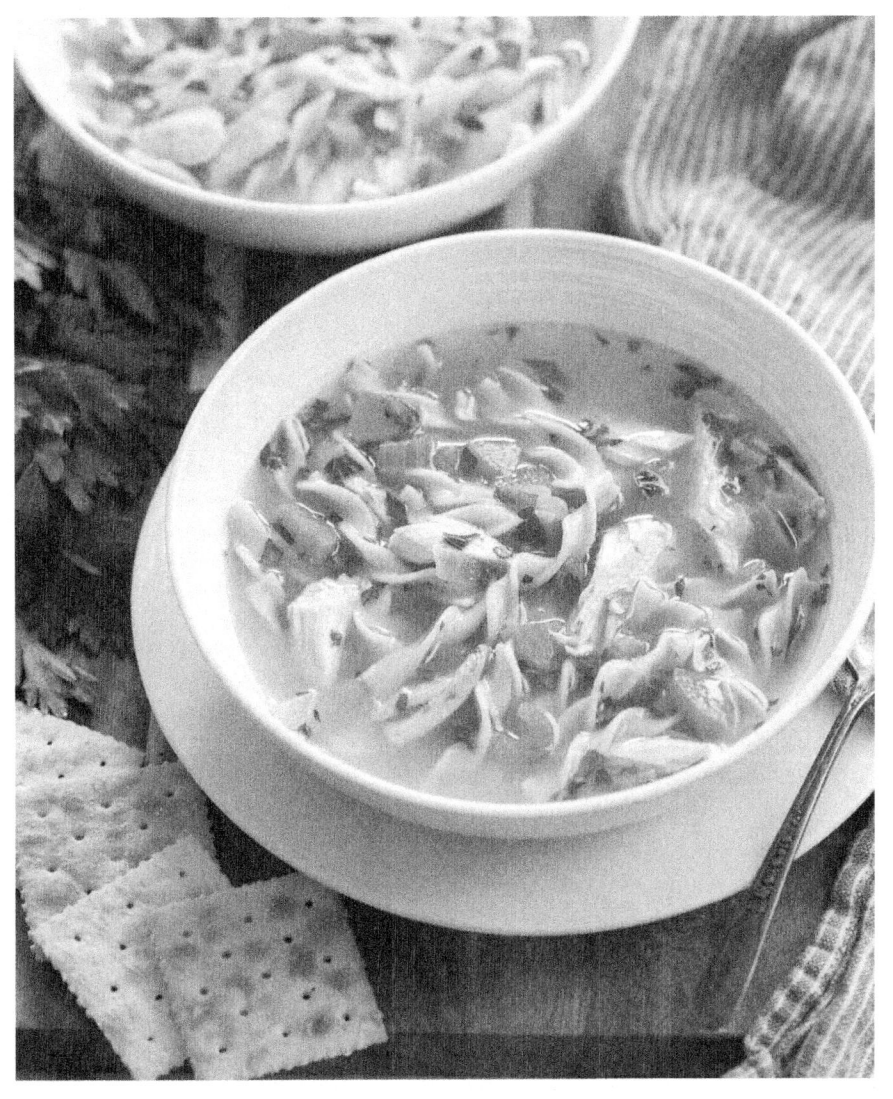

Homemade Chicken Broth:
1. Cut 1 onion, carrots, and celery into quarters (include the tops of the carrots and celery if you have them). Place the remaining ½ onion into the cavity of the chicken.
2. Place chicken in a large pot and add vegetables from step 1, fresh herbs, bay leaves, peppercorns, salt, and poultry seasoning. Cover with water.
3. Cover pot and bring to a boil over high heat. Once boiling, turn heat down and simmer partially covered for 1 ½ – 2 hours.
4. Remove chicken, shred meat and discard bones. Strain broth through cheesecloth. Discard the vegetables in the strainer (*see note 1).

Soup
1. Bring 8 cups of the strained broth to a boil and add carrots and celery. Cook 5 minutes.
2. While carrots are cooking, bring a pot of salted water to a boil. Cook egg noodles according to package directions. Drain and set aside. *see note 2
3. Stir in chicken and simmer until heated through, about 2 minutes. Season with salt and pepper to taste.
4. Place noodles in the bottom of each bowl. Ladle soup over top and serve.

NUTRITION FACTS

Calories: 138, Carbohydrates: 14g, Protein: 9g, Fat: 5g, Saturated Fat: 1g, Cholesterol: 31mg, Sodium: 1204mg, Potassium: 479mg, Fiber: 2g, Sugar: 2g, Vitamin A: 5459IU, Vitamin C: 25mg, Calcium: 44mg, Iron: 1mg

Vegetable Soup Recipe

PREP TIME: 10 minutes   **Serves:** 12
COOK TIME: 18 minutes
TOTAL TIME: 2 8 minutes

2

This Vegetable Soup Recipe is one of our favorites! Loaded with veggies and naturally low in fat and calories, it's the perfect lunch, snack, or starter!

- 1 teaspoon olive oil or butter
- 1 small onion diced
- 2 cloves garlic minced
- 4 cups cabbage chopped, approx. ¼ head of cabbage
- 1 cup carrots diced
- 1 cup green beans cut into 1" pieces
- 2 whole bell peppers chopped
- 2 cups cauliflower florets or broccoli
- 28 ounces low sodium diced tomatoes with juice
- 6 cups low sodium beef broth
- 2 tablespoons tomato paste
- 2 bay leaves
- ½ teaspoon thyme
- ½ teaspoon basil
- pepper to taste
- 2 cups zucchini sliced

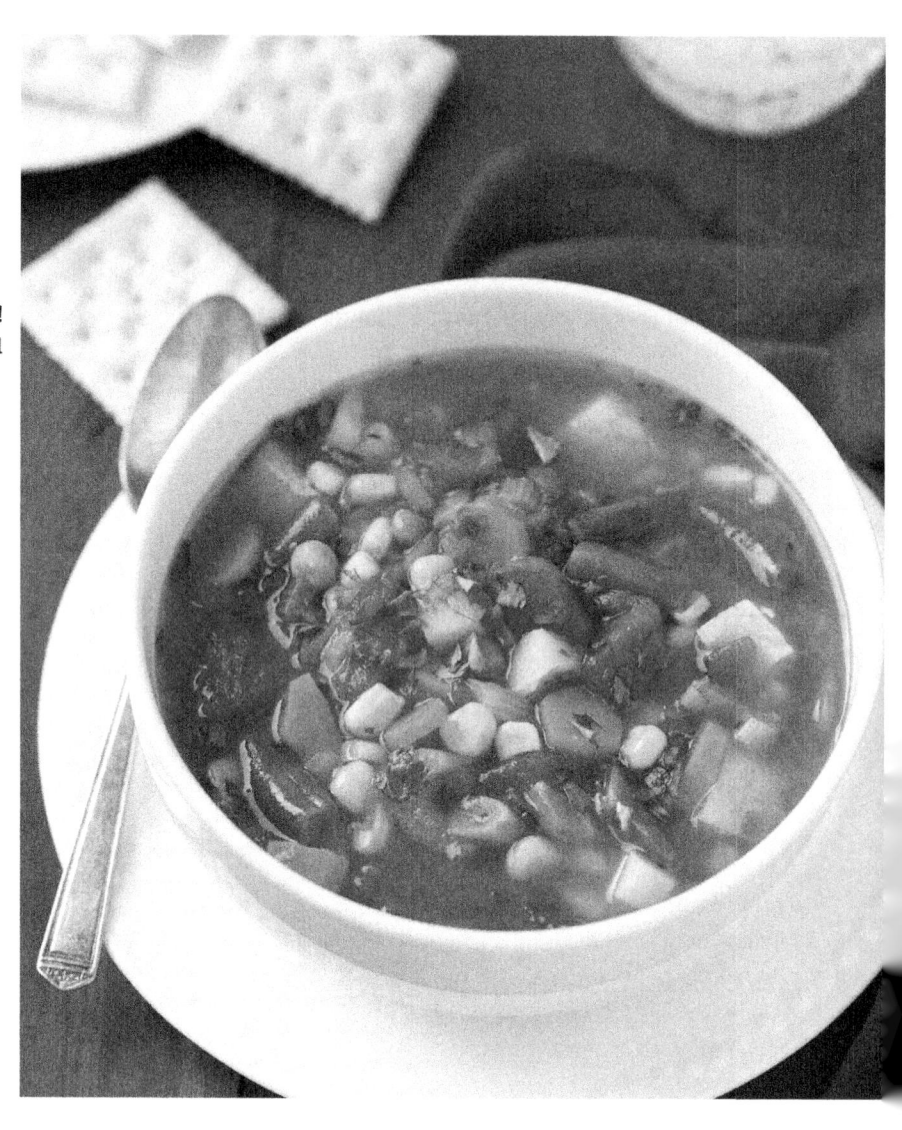

1. Heat olive oil in a large pot over medium heat. Add onion & garlic and cook until slightly softened, about 3 minutes.
2. Add cabbage, carrots, & green beans and cook for an additional 5 minutes.
3. Stir in bell peppers, cauliflower, undrained tomatoes, broth, tomato paste, bay leaves, and seasonings. Simmer 8-10 minutes.
4. Add in zucchini, simmer an additional 5 minutes or until softened.
5. Remove bay leaves before serving.

Recipe Notes:
1. Add any type of vegetables you'd like. Quick cooking veggies like spinach and zucchini should be added at the end of cooking.
2. To make a hearty meal, add in cooked protein before serving such as shredded chicken or ground beef. Whole grain pasta or rice can be added to each serving as well.
3. Optional flavor additions include: a few dashes of hot sauce, a sprinkle of parmesan cheese, fresh herbs.
4. Leftovers can be stored in an airtight container in the fridge for up to 4 days. Freeze cooled soup in individual portions for up to 4 months. Reheat or thaw directly on the stovetop.

NUTRITION FACTS

Serving: 1cup, Calories: 52, Carbohydrates: 10g, Protein: 4g, Fat: 1g, Saturated Fat: 1g, Polyunsaturated Fat: 1g, Monounsaturated Fat: 1g, Sodium: 268mg, Potassium: 646mg, Fiber: 3g, Sugar: 6g, Vitamin A: 2650IU, Vitamin C: 55mg, Calcium: 49mg, Iron: 1mg

Minestrone Soup

PREP TIME: 20 minutes   **Serves:** 6
COOK TIME: 30 minutes
TOTAL TIME: 50 minutes

5

This Minestrone Soup recipe is an easy one-pot meal that is full of vegetables, pasta, and an incredible tomato base. It's the perfect hearty dinner for a cool fall day!

- 1 tablespoon oil
- 3 large carrots finely chopped
- 2 stalks celery sliced
- ½ medium onion finely diced
- 1 teaspoon garlic minced
- 1 teaspoon dried parsley
- 1 teaspoon dried oregano
- 1 teaspoon dried basil
- ½ teaspoon salt
- ⅛ teaspoon black pepper
- 28 ounces canned diced tomatoes with juice
- 4 cups low sodium chicken broth
- 540 ml canned red kidney beans rinsed (about 2 cups)
- 1 ½ cups Rotini pasta dry
- 2 cups fresh spinach finely chopped
- Parmesan for serving, shredded or grated

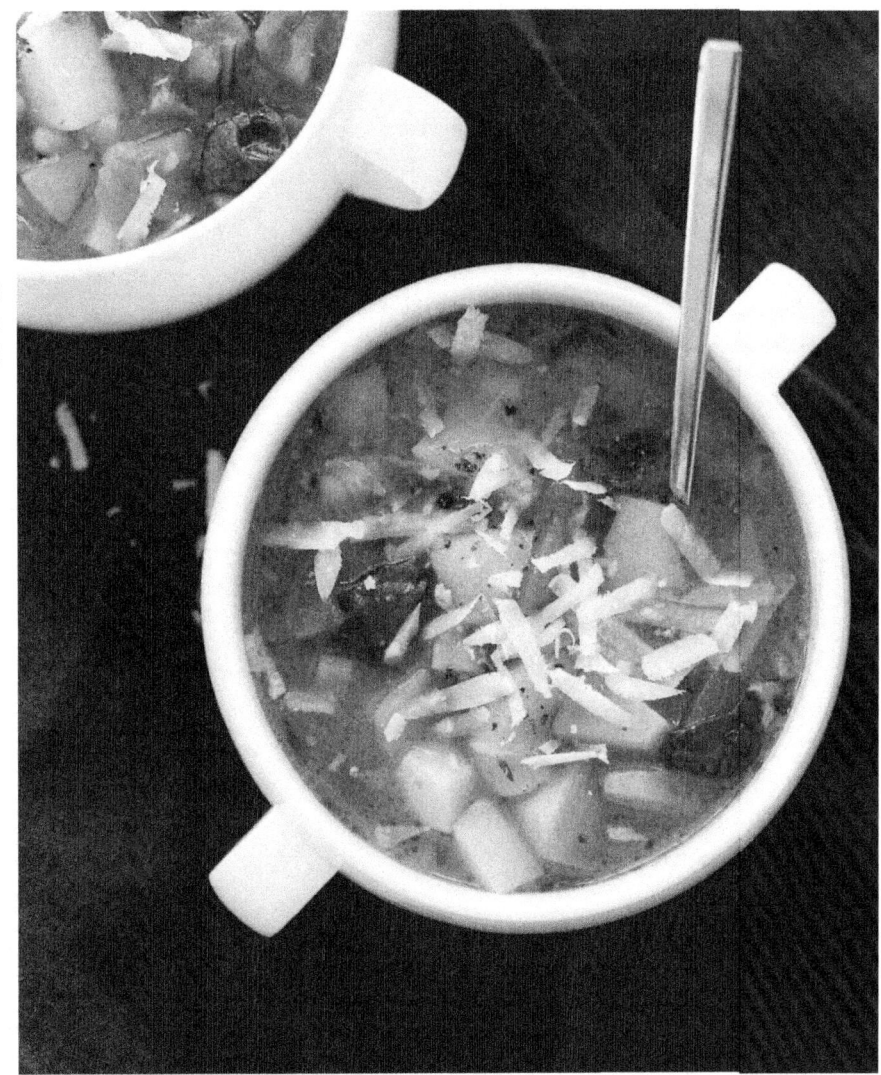

1. In a large pot cook and stir the oil, carrots, celery and onion over medium-high heat until the onion has softened, about 3-4 minutes.
2. Add the garlic, parsley, oregano, basil, salt, and pepper and cook for 1 minute.
3. Add the tomatoes, broth, and beans. Cover, bring to a boil and simmer over medium heat for 10-12 minutes or until carrots are tender.
4. Add the pasta and stir, cover, and simmer for 10 minutes or until pasta reaches desired tenderness. Stir in spinach and let sit for 2 minutes.
5. Serve with shredded Parmesan cheese as desired.

Recipe Notes:
1. IMPORTANT TIP: If you're planning for leftovers, cook the pasta separately and add it to each bowl individually. If pasta is cooked with the soup, it will get mushy if it sits in the fridge overnight or is frozen so drain it and store it separately. If cooking separately, be sure to salt the water or cook in broth for the best flavor.
2. You can substitute rice for pasta, you'll need about 2/3 cup uncooked rice.
3. You can mix and match your veggies as you wish. Keep it meatless or add in your own favorite protein like cooked Italian sausage.
4. This is a good soup for using up leftover veggies or, if time is short, use mixed frozen vegetables.
5. Always rinse canned beans in cold water to rinse off any preservatives and extra sodium.

NUTRITION FACTS

Calories: 219, Carbohydrates: 36g, Protein: 11g, Fat: 4g, Sodium: 1283mg, Potassium: 852mg, Fiber: 8g, Sugar: 7g, Vitamin A: 6250IU, Vitamin C: 18.9mg, Calcium: 113mg, Iron: 3.6mg

Homemade French Onion Soup

PREP TIME 15 minutes
COOK TIME 1 hour 20 minutes
TOTAL TIME 1 hour 35 minutes

Serves: 6

21

This flavorful French Onion Soup has rich beef broth filled with caramelized onions and topped with a golden bubbly cheese.

- 3 large sweet onions peeled
- ⅓ cup unsalted butter
- ½ teaspoon brown sugar optional
- 8 cups beef broth 64 oz
- ⅓ cup dry white wine
- 3 sprigs fresh thyme or ½ teaspoon dry
- 1 bay leaf
- ¼ teaspoon pepper
- 1 tablespoon Worcestershire sauce
- 1 tablespoon dry sherry optional
- 1 baguette
- 3 cups gruyere cheese
- 6 tablespoons fresh parmesan cheese

1. Slice onions ¼" thick. Cook onions, stirring occasionally, over low heat in melted butter (with sugar if using) until golden, about 30-45 minutes.
2. Add beef broth, wine, thyme, bay leaf, black pepper, Worcestershire, dry sherry. Bring to a boil, reduce heat and simmer for 1 hour. Remove bay leaf and thyme (if fresh) and discard.
3. Meanwhile, slice bread and brush with olive oil. Broil 2 minutes per side or until golden.
4. Ladle soup into ceramic bowls. Add 2 slices of bread to each bowl. Divide cheeses over bowls and broil until golden and bubbly.

Recipe Notes:

1. Choose sweet Vidalia or Walla Walla onions or yellow onions for this recipe. Sweeter varieties of onions may not need the sugar.
2. Onions will reduce down to a small amount but you'll need a large pan or dutch oven to begin.
3. Cook the onions very slowly, this step should take 30-40 minutes at a low temperature. This is where the flavor comes from.
4. For white wine choose a chardonnay, Pinot Gris, or Sauvignon Blanc. You can leave the wine out but it is recommended for the best flavor.
5. Leftover chunks of dry bread will work well as the bread in this recipe too.
6. Place the bowls on a baking sheet, this makes them easier to transfer in and out of the oven.
7. French onion soup freezes beautifully. Cook and cool the onions and broth and then place in freezer bags. Thaw in a pot on the stove until hot and then top with bread and cheese and broil.

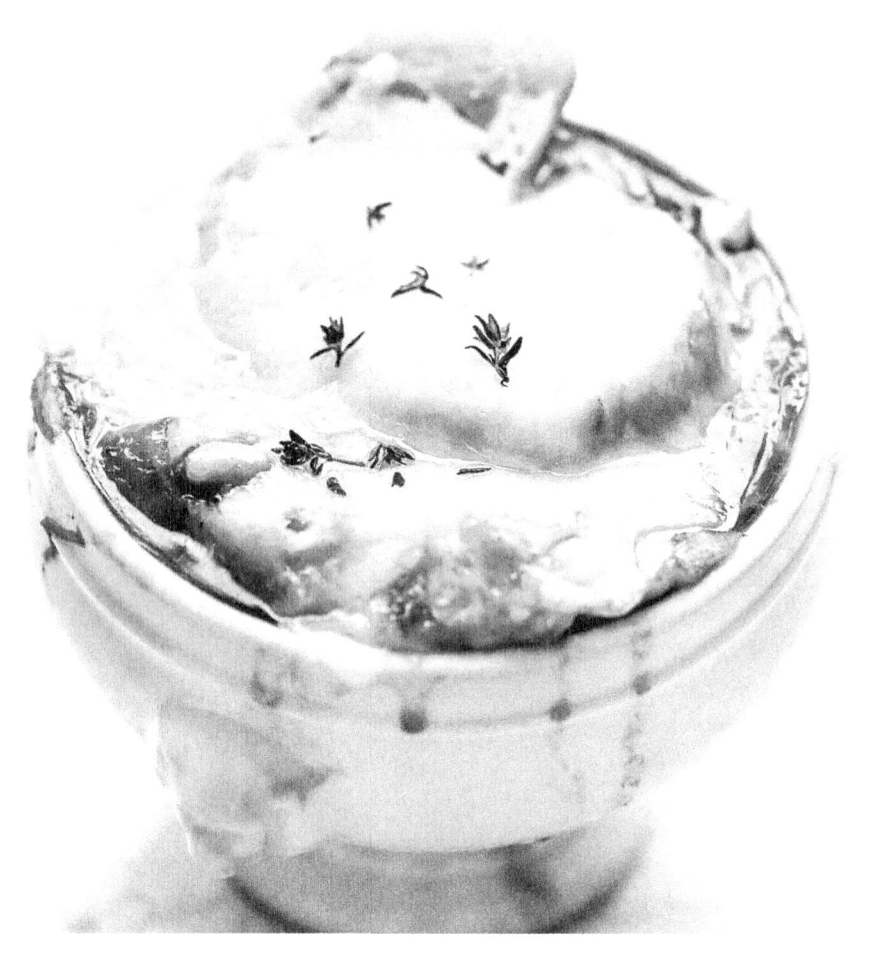

NUTRITION FACTS

Calories: 552, Carbohydrates: 27g, Protein: 31g, Fat: 34g, Saturated Fat: 20g, Cholesterol: 103mg, Sodium: 1264mg, Potassium: 851mg, Fiber: 2g, Sugar: 3g, Vitamin A: 1005IU, Vitamin C: 5.3mg, Calcium: 780mg, Iron: 1.8mg

Mac and Cheese Soup

PREP TIME: 15 minutes
COOK TIME: 15 minutes
TOTAL TIME: 30 minutes

Serves: 4

21

Creamy and delicious mac & cheese soup is loaded with 3 kinds of cheese.

- 4-5 cups chicken broth or stock see note
- 1 ¼ cup uncooked elbow macaroni

Cheese Base
- 2 tablespoons butter
- 2 tablespoons flour
- 2 cloves garlic minced
- 1 cup milk
- 4 ounces spreadable cream cheese
- 1 cup sharp cheddar cheese shredded
- ½ cup swiss cheese shredded, or additional cheddar cheese
- ½ teaspoon onion powder
- ½ teaspoon dry mustard
- ¼ teaspoon salt
- ¼ teaspoon pepper

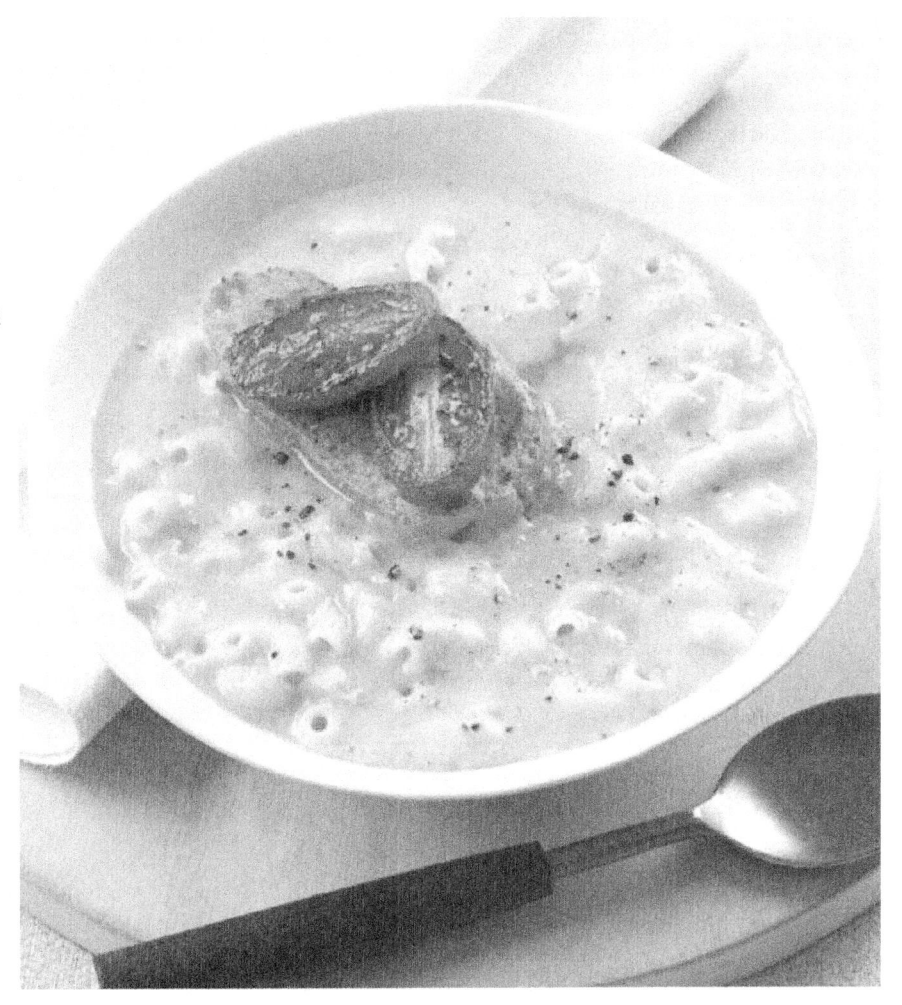

1. In a medium pot, bring the chicken broth to a boil. Add the elbow macaroni and cook until al dente, per the time indicated on the package. Do not drain.
2. While the pasta is cooking, melt butter in a separate saucepan and whisk in the flour. Cook for 1 minute.
3. Add garlic and cook until fragrant, about 30 seconds. Slowly whisk in milk a little at a time until smooth. Stir in seasonings and cook over medium heat while whisking until thick and bubbly. Let boil for about 1 minute.
4. Reduce the heat to medium-low and stir in cream cheese and shredded cheeses. Whisk until smooth; the mixture will be thick.
5. Once the pasta is cooked, add along with the chicken broth into the cheese mixture. Stir to combine. Heat over medium heat about 3 minutes or until hot.
6. Taste and season with salt & pepper if desired. Garnish with additional cheese and parsley to taste.

Recipe Notes:
1. Start with 4 cups of chicken broth. Depending on the brand of pasta, you may need a little bit more. The soup will thicken as is cools so more broth can be added if desired.
2. Any small pasta can be used in this recipe.
3. Shred your own cheeses, pre-shredded cheeses do not melt as well.
4. This recipe calls for spreadable cream cheese as it melts easier. If you have block cream cheese, add it once the milk is thickened before adding the cheddar and simmer until smooth. You can use a hand blender if needed.
5. Flavored spreadable cream cheese (such as herb and garlic) works well in this recipe.
6. Add ham, shredded chicken, or smoked sausage if desired.

NUTRITION FACTS

Calories: 518, Carbohydrates: 35g, Protein: 23g, Fat: 32g, Saturated Fat: 18g, Polyunsaturated Fat: 2g, Monounsaturated Fat: 9g, Trans Fat: 1g, Cholesterol: 97mg, Sodium: 773mg, Potassium: 431mg, Fiber: 1g, Sugar: 8g, Vitamin A: 1073IU, Vitamin C: 1mg, Calcium: 430mg, Iron: 1mg

Cheesy Potato Soup

PREP TIME: 15 minutes **Serves:** 4
COOK TIME: 15 minutes
TOTAL TIME: 30 minutes

`20`

This cheesy potato soup is super filling & flavorful, loaded with potatoes & 3 different kinds of cheese!

- 3 cups chicken broth or stock not low sodium
- ½ teaspoon onion powder
- ½ teaspoon dry mustard
- 1 pound baking potatoes peeled cut into 2" pieces

Cheese Base

- 1 tablespoon butter
- 2 cloves garlic minced
- 1 tablespoon flour
- 1 cup milk
- 4 ounces cream cheese softened and cut into small cubes
- 1 cup cheddar cheese shredded
- ½ cup Gruyere shredded
- ¼ teaspoon salt
- ¼ teaspoon pepper

1. In a medium pot, bring chicken broth and seasonings to a boil and add potatoes. Reduce to a simmer and cook until fork-tender, about 15 minutes. Once tender, mash slightly using a hand masher.*
2. While potatoes are simmering, melt butter and garlic in a medium saucepan just until fragrant. Stir in flour and cook 1 minute more.
3. Add milk a little at a time stirring after each addition until it is smooth. Once all of the milk is added bring to a boil over medium heat and cook until thick and bubbly. Stir in cream cheese and onion powder and whisk until smooth.
4. Turn off the heat and add shredded cheese. Stir until melted.
5. Combine the smashed potato mixture and the cheese mixture. Add the potato broth to reach desired consistency (I usually use all of it).
6. Simmer 1 minute to combine. Season with additional salt and pepper to taste and garnish as desired.

Recipe Notes:

1. We love Russet potatoes for this recipe but other potatoes will work. If using red or Yukon gold potatoes, peeling is optional.
2. *Mash the potatoes to desired consistency. The more you mash, the thicker the soup will be.
3. When adding the cream cheese, I like to use a hand blender to make it smooth.
4. Do not overheat the cheese or it can separate.
5. Garnish as desired. Favorites include sour cream, chives, thyme, green onion, crumbled bacon, croutons or breadsticks.

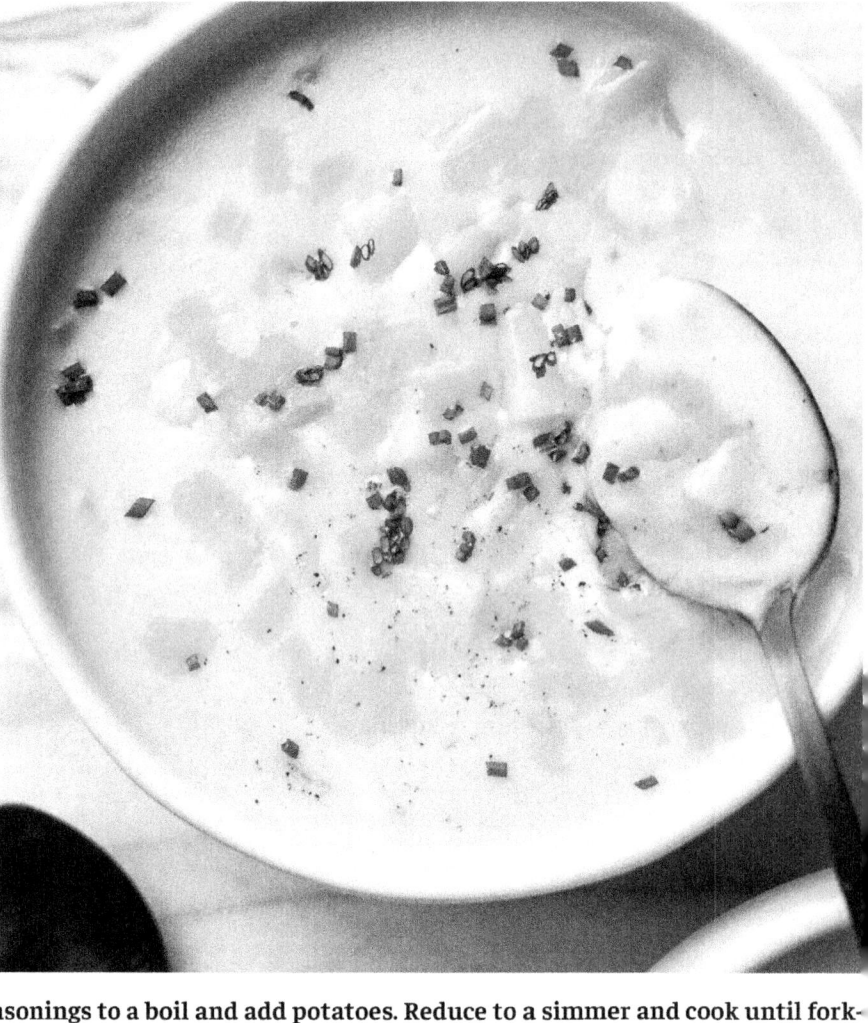

NUTRITION FACTS

Calories: 494, Carbohydrates: 33g, Protein: 23g, Fat: 30g, Saturated Fat: 17g, Polyunsaturated Fat: 2g, Monounsaturated Fat: 9g, Trans Fat: 1g, Cholesterol: 95mg, Sodium: 782mg, Potassium: 843mg, Fiber: 2g, Sugar: 8g, Vitamin A: 1031IU, Vitamin C: 7mg, Calcium: 497mg, Iron: 2mg

Ham Bone Soup (Slow Cooker)

PREP TIME: 5 minutes
COOK TIME: 6 hours
TOTAL TIME: 6 hours 5 minutes
Serves: 8

21

A ham bone is slow cooked with veggies like potatoes, carrots, corn, and beans. Serve it with some easy dinner rolls for the perfect meal!

- 1 meaty ham bone
- 1 pound Yukon gold potatoes diced
- 3 carrots sliced
- 2 ribs celery sliced
- 1 cup corn
- 1 large onion diced
- 15 ounces cannellini beans drained and rinsed (white kidney beans)
- 7 cups chicken broth or water
- 2 bay leaves
- 2 sprigs thyme or 1 teaspoon dried thyme leaves
- ¼ cup fresh parsley

1. Combine all ingredients in the slow cooker.
2. Cover soup and cook on high 6 hours or low 9-10 hours.
3. Remove ham bone, bay leaves and thyme stems (if using fresh thyme).
4. Chop meat from the bone and add back into the soup. Stir and serve.

Recipe Notes:
1. The size of your ham bone or the amount of meat on the bone can add more or less flavor.

NUTRITION FACTS

Per Serving:: Calories: 349, Carbohydrates: 60g, Protein: 19g, Fat: 5g, Saturated Fat: 1g, Polyunsaturated Fat: 2g, Monounsaturated Fat: 2g, Trans Fat: 1g, Sodium: 1080mg, Potassium: 1317mg, Fiber: 12g, Sugar: 9g, Vitamin A: 7210IU, Vitamin C: 23mg, Calcium: 175mg, Iron: 6mg

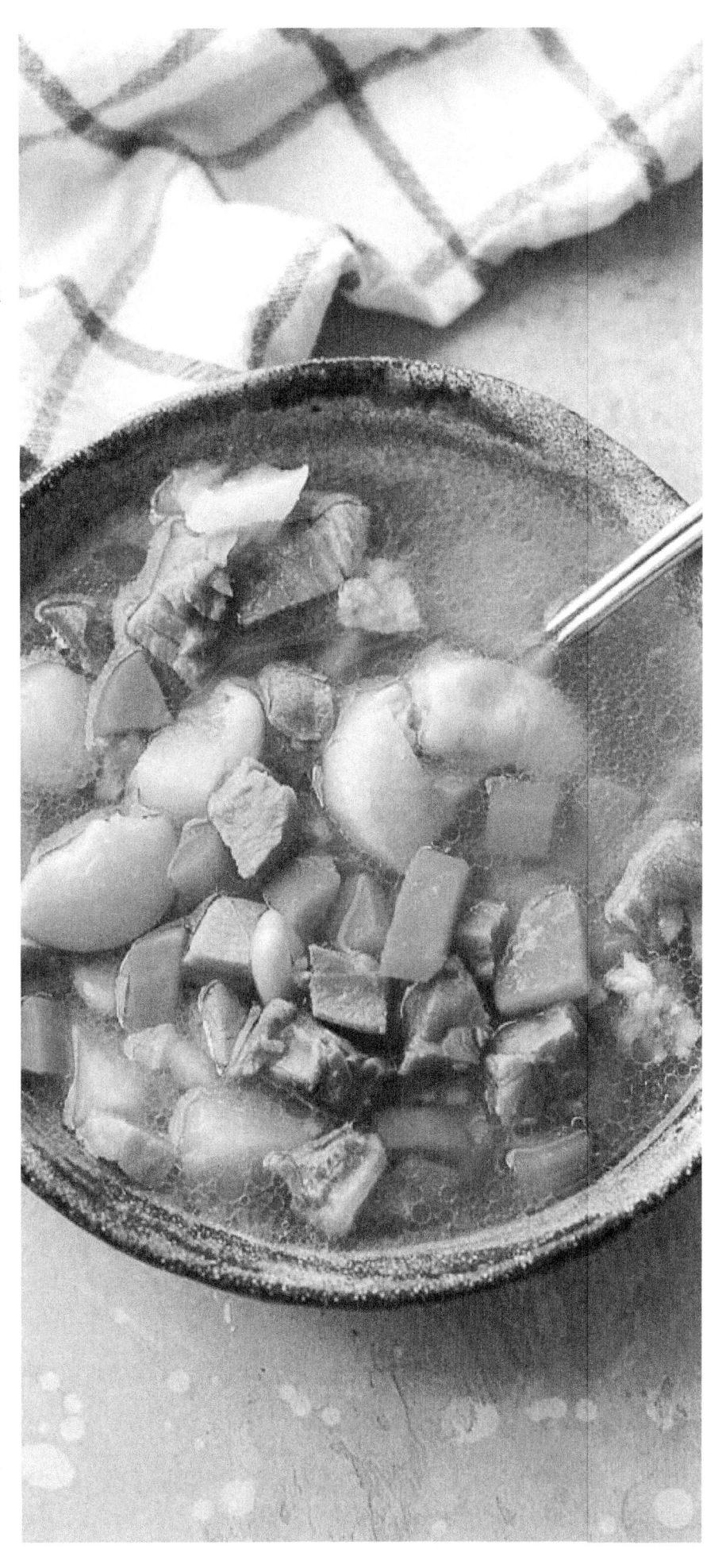

Quick Cabbage Soup

PREP TIME: 15 minutes   Serves: 8
COOK TIME: 30 minutes
TOTAL TIME: 45 minutes

4

This healthy & budget-friendly soup is so easy to make and freezes well for quick lunch or dinners!

- 2 teaspoons olive oil
- ½ onion diced
- 6 cups cabbage
- 14 ounces diced tomatoes with juice
- 6 cups beef broth or chicken broth
- 1 carrot shredded
- 1 tablespoon tomato paste
- 1 tablespoon parsley fresh
- 1 teaspoon Italian seasoning
- 1 bay leaf

1. Cook onion in olive oil until tender, 3-4 minutes.
2. While onion is cooking, dice cabbage into ½" pieces. Add cabbage to the pot and cook over medium heat until it starts to soften, about 8 minutes.
3. While cabbage is cooking prepare other ingredients. Add all ingredients to the pot, bring to a boil and simmer uncovered 15 minutes or until cabbage is tender.
4. Discard bay leaf, season with salt & pepper to taste and serve.

Recipe Notes:
1. Leftover soup can be stored in the fridge for up to 4 days.
2. Freeze cooled soup in individual portions for up to 2 months.
3. Reheat in the microwave or in a pot on the stovetop.

NUTRITION FACTS

Calories: 189, Carbohydrates: 22g, Protein: 13g, Fat: 6g, Saturated Fat: 2g, Cholesterol: 21mg, Sodium: 574mg, Potassium: 512mg, Fiber: 5g, Sugar: 3g, Vitamin A: 4070IU, Vitamin C: 13.3mg, Calcium: 75mg, Iron: 3.6mg

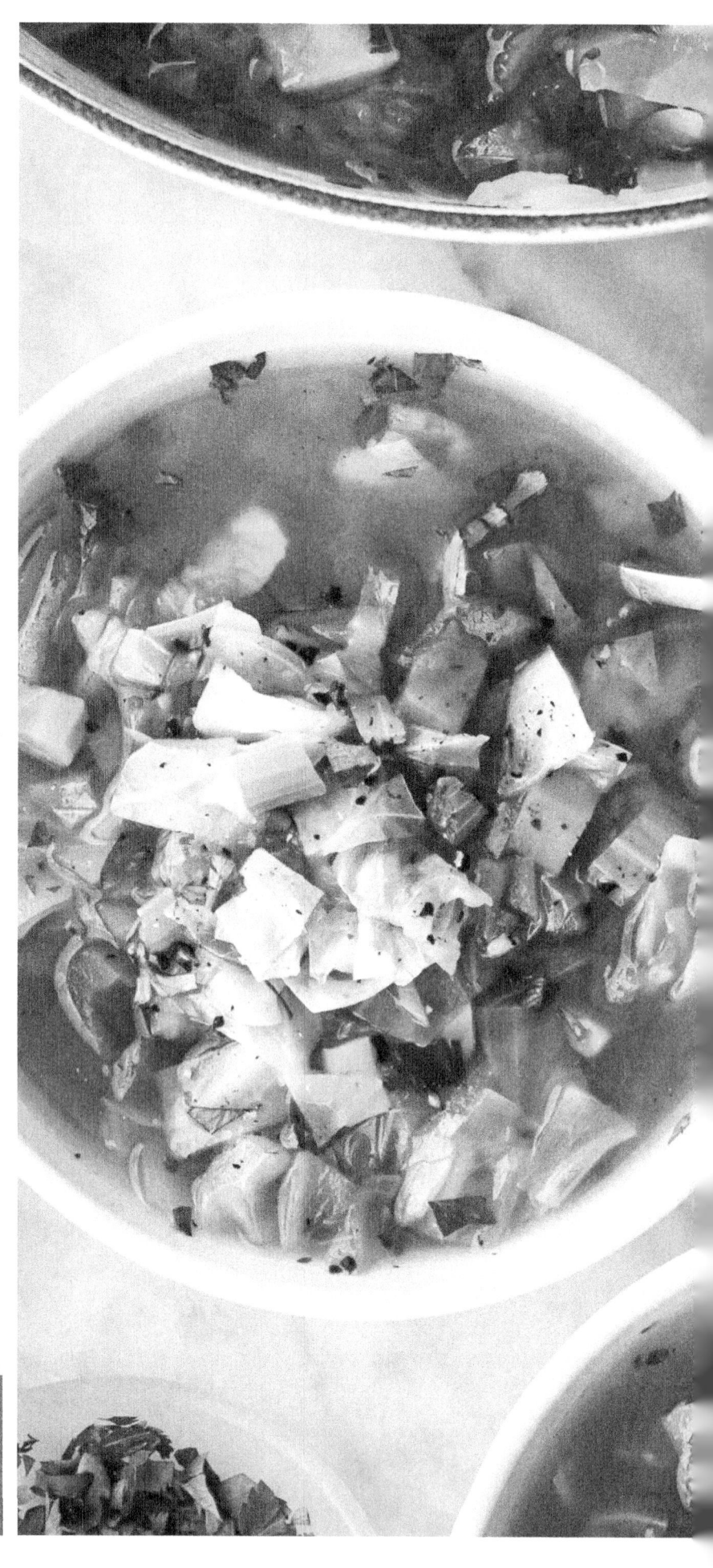

Chapter 3:
Dessert

Homemade Cinnamon Roll Recipe

PREP TIME: 20 minutes **Serves:** 15
COOK TIME: 2 hours 30 minutes
TOTAL TIME: 2 hours 50 minutes

17

This recipe makes soft rolls with sticky-sweet cinnamon filling on the inside, and dripping with cream cheese icing on the outside!

- ¼ cup warm water
- 1 package active dry yeast or 2 ¼ teaspoons
- ¾ cup whole milk
- ⅓ cup butter
- ⅓ cup granulated sugar plus 1 teaspoon
- ½ teaspoon salt
- 3 ¾ to 4 ¼ cups all purpose flour divided
- 2 eggs room temperature

Filling
- ½ cup butter softened
- 1 cup brown sugar packed
- 2 tablespoons ground cinnamon

Frosting
- 1 ½ cups powdered sugar or as needed
- 4 ounces cream cheese softened
- ¼ cup unsalted butter softened
- ½ teaspoon vanilla extract
- ⅛ teaspoon salt

1. Grease a 9x13 pan or baking dish.
2. Combine water, yeast, and 1 teaspoon sugar in a small bowl. Let sit 10 minutes or until foamy.
3. Combine milk, butter, remaining sugar, and salt in a saucepan and heat to 120-130°F.
4. Place 2 cups flour in a stand mixer. Add eggs, milk mixture, and yeast mixture. Mix until combined.
5. Using a dough hook, add flour, ½ cup at a time, to form a soft dough that pulls away from the side of the bowl. Remove dough from the bowl and knead on a lightly floured surface until dough is smooth and elastic (approx. 8 mins).
6. Place in a greased bowl in a warm spot and cover with a towel for 1 hour or until doubled in size.
7. Roll dough into a 15" x 12" rectangle, spread butter on the dough and top with brown sugar and cinnamon.
8. Roll dough starting on the long side. Slice into 15 pieces. Place in prepared pan.
9. Cover rolls with a towel and allow them to rise 30-45 minutes. Preheat oven to 375°F.
10. Brush rolls with milk and bake 20-25 minutes.
11. While the rolls are baking, combine powdered sugar, cream cheese, butter, vanilla extract, and salt with a mixer until fluffy.
12. Allow rolls to cool for about 10-15 minutes and spread frosting on warm rolls.

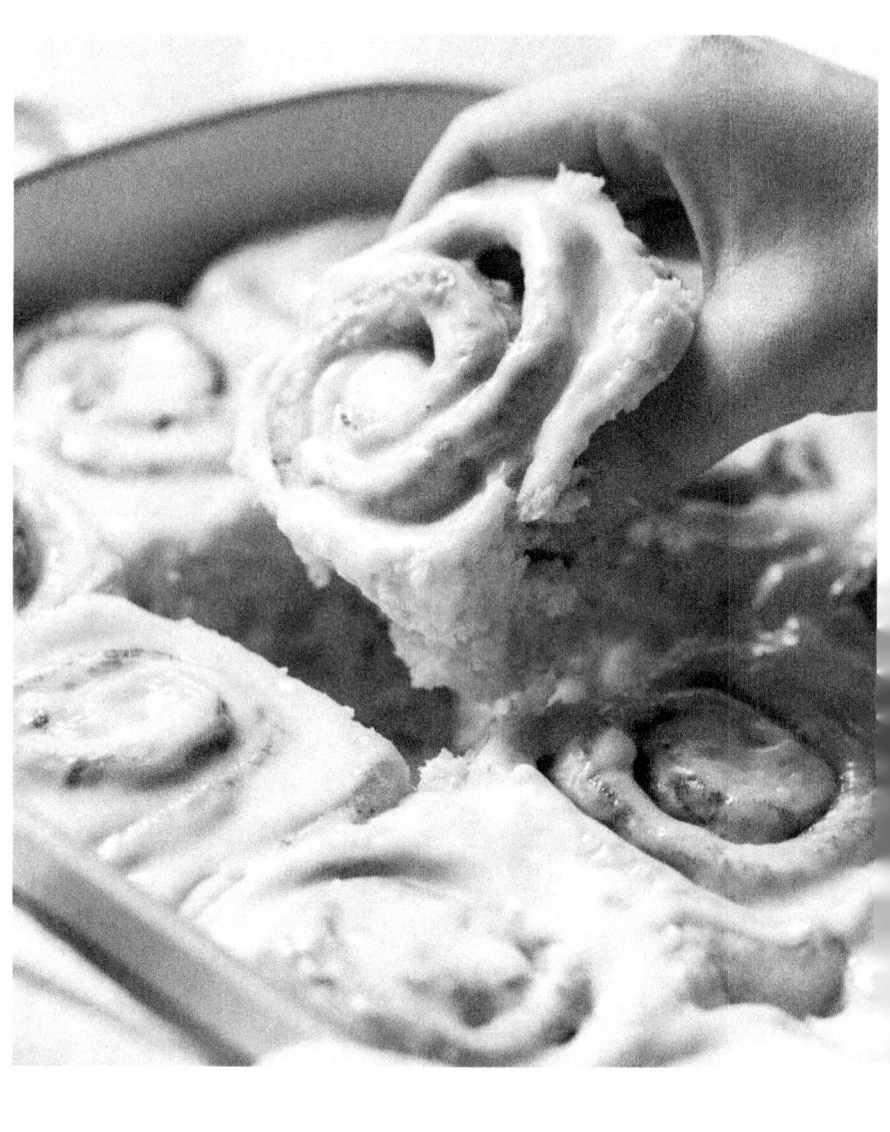

NUTRITION FACTS

Calories: 406, Carbohydrates: 59g, Protein: 6g, Fat: 17g, Saturated Fat: 10g, Cholesterol: 66mg, Sodium: 257mg, Potassium: 103mg, Fiber: 2g, Sugar: 30g, Vitamin A: 566IU, Calcium: 58mg, Iron: 2mg

Peanut Butter Cake

PREP TIME: 20 minutes　　**Serves:** 15
COOK TIME: 40 minutes
TOTAL TIME: 1 hour

31

Peanut Butter Cake is sweet and fluffy with homemade creamy frosting on top. It's sure to be a treat the whole family will love.

Cake:
- 3 cups cake flour
- 1 tablespoon baking powder
- 1 teaspoon salt
- 1 ¾ cups light brown sugar packed
- ½ cup unsalted butter softened
- ½ cup vegetable oil
- 2 teaspoons vanilla extract
- ¾ cup creamy peanut butter
- 4 large eggs
- 1 ¼ cups whole milk

Frosting:
- 1 cup unsalted butter softened
- 1 cup creamy peanut butter
- ¼ cup unsweetened cocoa powder
- 3 cups powdered sugar
- ¼ cup heavy cream

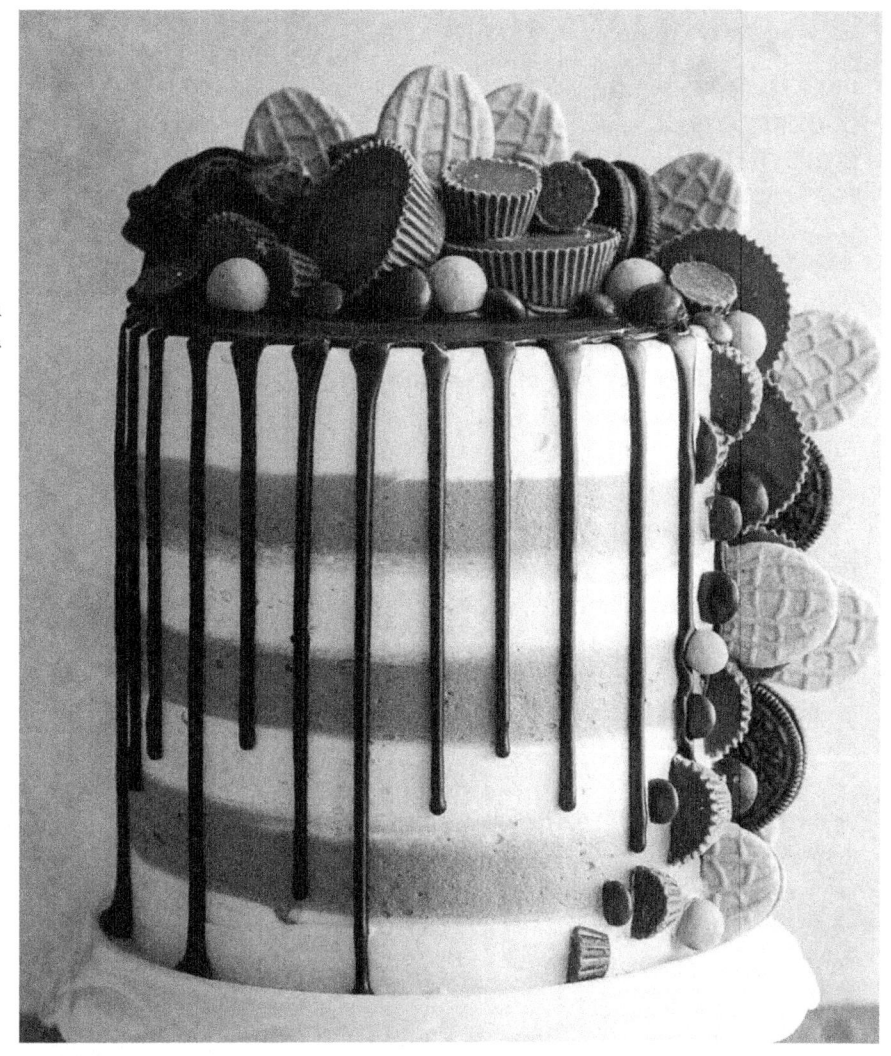

1. Preheat oven to 350°F. Grease and flour a 9x13 pan.
2. Place cake flour, baking powder, and salt in a bowl and whisk to combine.
3. With an electric mixer or stand mixer on medium speed, cream brown sugar and butter until fluffy. Add oil and vanilla and mix until combined.
4. Increase the speed to medium-high and beat until light and fluffy, 3-4 minutes.
5. Add peanut butter and mix until incorporated and then add eggs one at a time.
6. Alternate adding flour and milk a bit at a time just until incorporated. Be sure not to overmix.
7. Spread the batter into the prepared baking pan. Bake 28-32 minutes or until a toothpick comes out clean.
8. Remove from the oven and allow to cool completely before frosting.

To Frost:
1. While the cake is baking, cream butter and peanut butter.
2. Add cocoa powder and mix until fully incorporated.
3. Add powdered sugar 1 cup at a time, mixing slowly until incorporated.
4. Slowly add in the heavy cream with the mixer running on low speed until incorporated then increase speed to medium-high and whip for about 2 minutes until light and fluffy.
5. Once cooled spread the frosting over the cake and serve.

NUTRITION FACTS

Calories: 735, Carbohydrates: 76g, Protein: 13g, Fat: 45g, Saturated Fat: 18g, Polyunsaturated Fat: 6g, Monounsaturated Fat: 19g, Trans Fat: 1g, Cholesterol: 99mg, Sodium: 321mg, Potassium: 389mg, Fiber: 3g, Sugar: 53g, Vitamin A: 722IU, Vitamin C: 1mg, Calcium: 116mg, Iron: 1mg

Strawberry Pretzel Salad

PREP TIME: 20 minutes
COOK TIME: 15 minutes
CHILL TIME: 6 hours
TOTAL TIME: 6 hours 35 minutes

Serves: 12

Strawberry Pretzel Salad is a classic family favorite dessert. This easy make-ahead recipe is the most delicious combo of sweet and salty, creamy and crunchy!

Pretzel Crust
- 2 cups crushed pretzels
- ¾ cup butter melted
- 3 tablespoons sugar

Creamy Filling
- 8 ounces cream cheese softened
- ¾ cup sugar
- 8 ounces Cool Whip defrosted

Strawberry Topping
- 6 ounces Strawberry Jell-O
- 2 cups boiling water
- 4 cups sliced strawberries

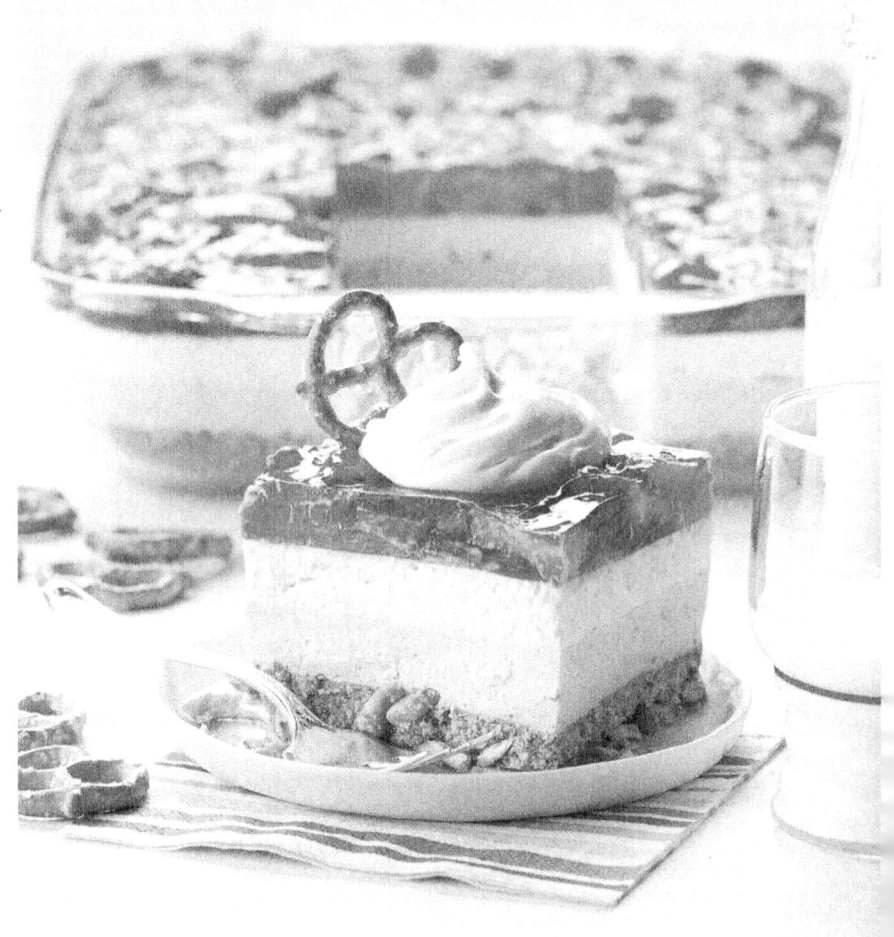

1. Preheat oven to 375°F.
2. Combine crushed pretzels, butter, and sugar in a bowl and press into the bottom of a 9x13 pan. Bake 10 minutes and cool completely.
3. In a medium bowl, mix cream cheese and sugar with a hand mixer on medium until fluffy. Gently fold in Cool Whip. Spread mixture evenly over the cooled crust and refrigerate at least 1 hour.
4. In a large mixing bowl combine Jell-O and boiling water until jello is dissolved. Allow mixture to sit at room temperature until completely cooled.
5. Place sliced strawberries over the cream cheese mixture. Pour cooled Jell-O overtop.
6. Refrigerate until firmly set, at least 4-6 hours or overnight.

Recipe Notes:
1. Do not follow the instructions on the Jell-o box. Ensure the Jell-o is the larger 6 oz size box.
2. The pretzels are crushed first and then measured.
3. For easy removal from the pan, the dish can be lined with parchment paper.

NUTRITION FACTS

Calories: 244, Carbohydrates: 34g, Protein: 1g, Fat: 12g, Saturated Fat: 7g, Cholesterol: 30mg, Sodium: 274mg, Potassium: 94mg, Fiber: 1g, Sugar: 22g, Vitamin A: 360IU, Vitamin C: 28.2mg, Calcium: 15mg, Iron: 0.9mg

Toll House Cookie Recipe

PREP TIME: 10 minutes **Serves:** 48
COOK TIME: 10 minutes
TOTAL TIME: 20 minutes

6

Chewy on the inside and crispy on the outside, buttery-flavored chocolate chip cookies just melt in your mouth!

- 2 ¼ cups all-purpose flour
- 1 teaspoon baking soda
- 1 teaspoon salt
- 1 cup butter softened
- ¾ cup granulated sugar
- ¾ cup packed brown sugar
- 1 teaspoon vanilla extract
- 2 large eggs
- 2 cups Toll House Semi-Sweet Chocolate Morsels 12 oz package
- 1 cup chopped nuts Optional. If omitting, add 1 to 2 Tbsp. of all-purpose flour.

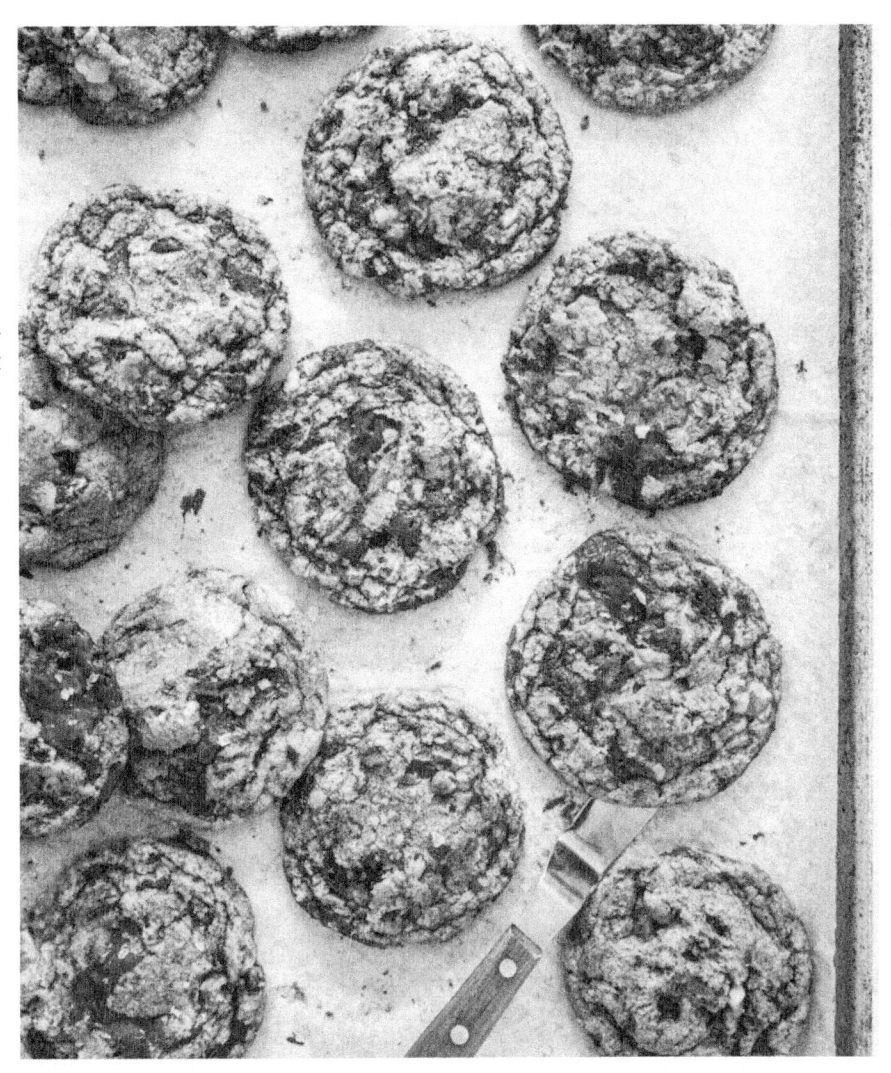

1. Preheat oven to 375°F.
2. Place flour, salt, and baking soda in a bowl and mix with a whisk or fork. Set aside.
3. Which a hand mixer on medium speed, combine butter, brown and white sugar, and vanilla. Beat until creamy, about 2 minutes.
4. Add eggs in one at a time and beat after each addition. Once incorporated, add in the flour mixture a bit at a time until combined.
5. Stir in the chocolate chips with a spoon and chill the dough in the fridge for 30 minutes. Drop by large tablespoons onto an ungreased baking sheet.
6. Bake 9-11 minutes or until lightly browned on the edges, do not over bake.
7. Allow the cookies to cool on the cookie sheet 2-3 minutes and then remove and cool on a wire rack.

Recipe Notes:
1. The chilling step can be skipped, the cookies will spread a little bit more but still be delicious.
2. Ensure ingredients are room temperature ingredients.
3. Use unsalted butter or omit the salt if using salted butter.
4. Ensure cookies are not placed on a warm pan or they will spread too much.
5. Avoid overcrowding the pan so the heat can circulate around each cookie.
6. Chill the dough before scooping and baking for a thicker cookie. This keeps them from flattening out too much and ensures a chewy interior.

NUTRITION FACTS

Serving: 1cookie, Calories: 143, Carbohydrates: 15g, Protein: 2g, Fat: 9g, Saturated Fat: 4g, Polyunsaturated Fat: 1g, Monounsaturated Fat: 2g, Trans Fat: 1g, Cholesterol: 18mg, Sodium: 110mg, Potassium: 68mg, Fiber: 1g, Sugar: 9g, Vitamin A: 134IU, Vitamin C: 1mg, Calcium: 13mg, Iron: 1mg

Homemade Brownies

PREP TIME: 15 minutes
COOK TIME: 25 minutes
TOTAL TIME: 40 minutes

Serves: 16

10

These Homemade Brownies are perfectly decadent, delicious, and loaded with chocolate chips!

- ½ cup butter melted
- 2 tablespoons vegetable oil
- 1 ⅓ cups sugar
- ⅔ cup unsweetened cocoa powder
- 2 large eggs room temperature
- 1 teaspoon vanilla extract
- 1 teaspoon espresso powder or instant coffee
- ½ teaspoon salt
- ½ cup flour
- 1 cup semi-sweet chocolate chips plus more for topping

1. Preheat oven to 350°F. Line a 9x9 pan with foil and coat with cooking spray.
2. Combine melted butter, oil, sugar, and cocoa powder in a large bowl. Stir until smooth.
3. Mix in the eggs, vanilla, espresso powder, and salt.
4. Slowly stir in the flour (batter should be thick) and gently fold in the chocolate chips.
5. Spread the batter into the prepared pan & top with more chocolate chips if desired.
6. Bake for 21-25 minutes or until they become glossy around the edges and a toothpick comes out clean when inserted 1-inch from the edge.
7. Let cool before cutting.

Recipe Notes:
1. For quick and easy clean-up, line the baking dish with parchment paper or foil. This also allows for you to easily remove and cut brownies by lifting them out.
2. Ensure eggs are room temperature, you can put them in a glass of warm water if you've forgotten to take them out early.
3. Do not overcook, brownies should be cooked until a toothpick 1-inch from the edge of the pan comes out with just a few crumbs attached. They can and should be a little bit gooey in the middle.
4. Make sure the brownies are completely cooled before cutting.
5. Line the pan with foil first, this makes the brownies easy to lift out before cutting.
6. Use a plastic knife if you have one, the brownies won't stick to a plastic knife. A regular knife can be sprayed with oil or cooking spray before cutting the brownies.

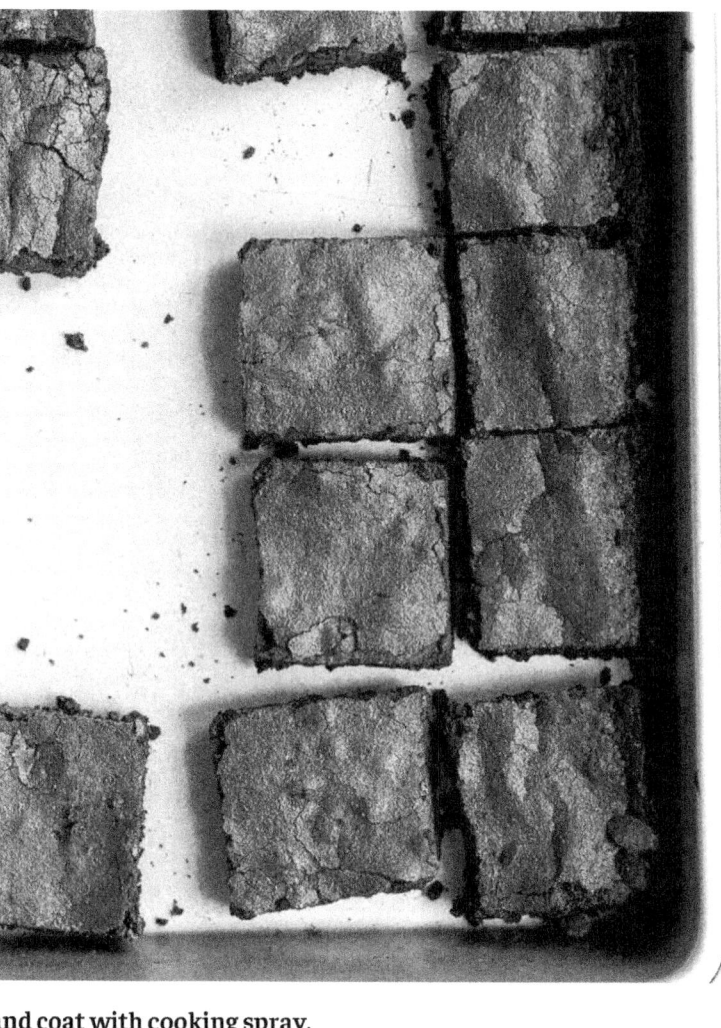

NUTRITION FACTS

Calories: 227, Carbohydrates: 28g, Protein: 3g, Fat: 13g, Saturated Fat: 7g, Polyunsaturated Fat: 1g, Monounsaturated Fat: 4g, Trans Fat: 1g, Cholesterol: 36mg, Sodium: 133mg, Potassium: 135mg, Fiber: 2g, Sugar: 21g, Vitamin A: 213IU, Calcium: 17mg, Iron: 2mg

Easy Red Velvet Cheesecake

PREP TIME: 10 minutes   Serves: 12
COOK TIME: 4 hours 20 minutes

25

This simple recipe combines Red Velvet cake and cheesecake for an impressive looking dessert that is super easy to make! A simple Red Velvet cake layer is topped with a deliciously quick and rich no bake cheesecake layer!

Red Velvet Cake
- 1 box red velvet cake mix 15.25 oz
- 1 egg
- ½ cup vegetable oil
- ⅓ cup milk

No Bake Cheesecake
- 12 ounces cream cheese
- 1 ½ cups powdered sugar
- 1 teaspoon vanilla
- 1 ½ cups heavy cream

Optional
- whipped cream & raspberries for decorating

1. Preheat oven to 350°F. Grease the bottom and sides of a 10" springform pan.
2. Combine dry cake mix, egg, oil and milk. Mix on medium 2 minutes or until smooth.
3. Spread into prepared pan and bake 20-25 minutes or until a toothpick comes out clean. Do not overbake. If needed gently press the edges with a spatula to even and flatten out the cake. Cool completely.
4. Beat together cream cheese, powdered sugar, and vanilla until fluffy. Add in heavy cream and continue beating until thick and creamy and stiff peaks form.
5. Run a butter knife around the edges of the red velvet cake to loosen it. Spread cheesecake mixture over the cooled red velvet cake. Cover and refrigerate 4 hours or overnight.
6. Decorate as desired.

Recipe Notes:
1. Be sure to follow the recipe below and do not follow the instructions on the back of the cake mix box!
2. Ensure that the cake layer is completely cooled or it will melt the cheesecake layer.
3. If you don't have a springform pan, line a 9" pan with parchment paper so it is easy to remove the cake and cut.
4. Once the cake layer is baked, gently press the edges with a spatula to even and flatten out the cake.
5. Be sure to refrigerate at least 4 hours. This cake freezes well and can be made ahead of time.

NUTRITION FACTS

Calories: 499, Carbohydrates: 44g, Protein: 5g, Fat: 36g, Saturated Fat: 21g, Cholesterol: 86mg, Sodium: 408mg, Potassium: 195mg, Fiber: 1g, Sugar: 30g, Vitamin A: 851IU, Vitamin C: 1mg, Calcium: 111mg, Iron: 2mg

No Churn Grape Ice Cream

PREP TIME: 5 minutes **Serves:** 8
COOK TIME: 15 minutes
CHILL TIME: 4 hours
TOTAL TIME: 4 hours 20 minutes

`19`

Infused with sweet grape jelly & pieces of plump grapes, this no-churn ice cream is rich, creamy, and so delicious!

- 1 cup finely chopped purple grapes
- 14 ounces sweetened condensed milk
- 2 teaspoons grape flavoring
- 2 cups heavy cream
- ¼ cup grape jelly optional

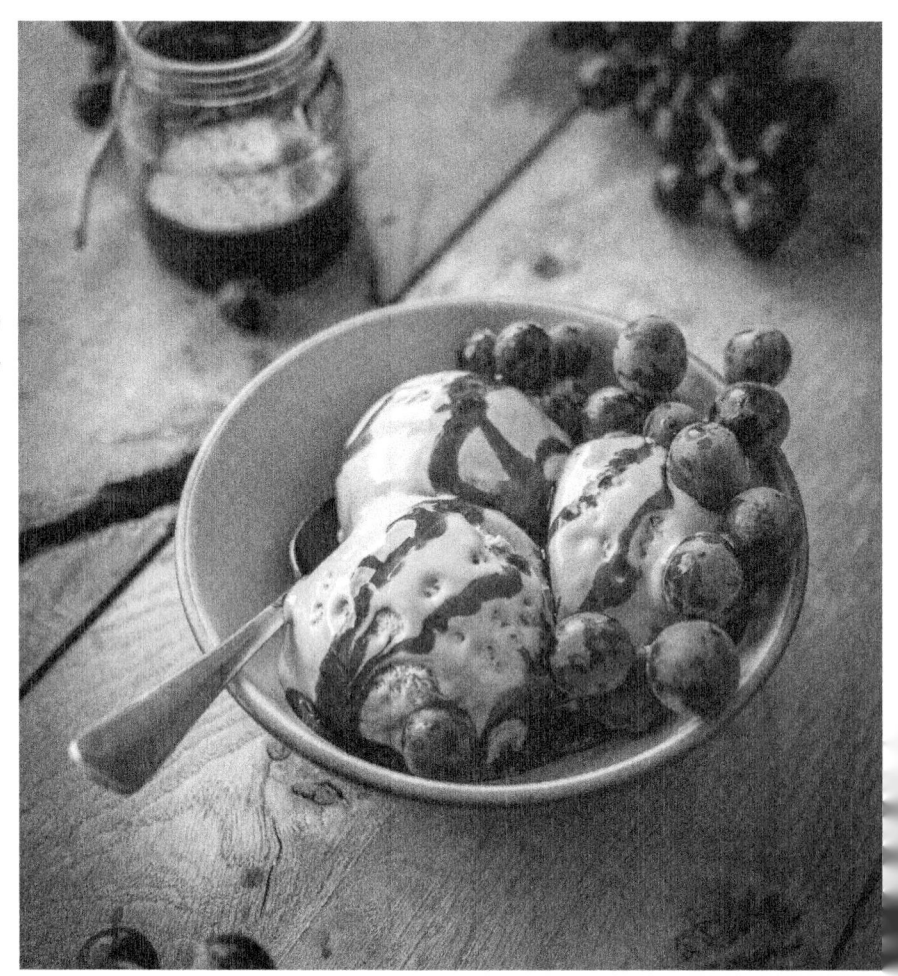

1. Line a 9x5 loaf pan with parchment paper. Place in the freezer along with two large mixing bowls for steps 3 & 4.
2. Wash grapes and pat dry. Chop into small pieces and place on a double layer of paper towel. Press gently to remove any liquid.
3. Combine sweetened condensed milk and grape flavoring in a large chilled bowl.
4. In the other chilled bowl, whip heavy cream on medium-high until stiff peaks form.
5. Gently fold the whipped cream into the sweetened condensed milk. Fold in grapes.
6. Place grape jelly in a bowl and whisk until slightly smooth. Place in a zip-top bag and snip off a small corner.
7. Spread half of the ice cream mixture into the prepared pan. Squeeze half of the jelly over the ice cream mixture. Top with the remaining ice cream mixture and drizzle with the remaining jelly. Swirl with a knife.
8. Cover with plastic wrap and freeze for at least 4 hours or overnight.

Recipe Notes:
1. Place the bowl and pan in the freezer while preparing the ingredients.
2. I have only made this recipe as written with grape flavoring, although the base does make a great vanilla ice cream with added vanilla extract. If you don't have grape flavoring you could try adding other flavorings or extracts however this will change the flavor of the recipe.
3. Store ice cream in an airtight container in the freezer for up to 2 weeks.

NUTRITION FACTS

Calories: 407, Carbohydrates: 39g, Protein: 5g, Fat: 26g, Saturated Fat: 16g, Polyunsaturated Fat: 1g, Monounsaturated Fat: 8g, Cholesterol: 98mg, Sodium: 89mg, Potassium: 273mg, Fiber: 1g, Sugar: 35g, Vitamin A: 1020IU, Vitamin C: 3mg, Calcium: 184mg, Iron: 1mg

Candied Pecans

PREP TIME: 10 minutes
COOK TIME: 40 minutes
TOTAL TIME: 50 minutes

Serves: 16

13

These candied pecans are easy to make and the perfect addition to salads, desserts or just for snacking!

- 1 cup white sugar
- 1 teaspoon ground cinnamon
- 1 teaspoon salt
- 1 egg white
- 1 tablespoon water
- 1 lb pecan halves

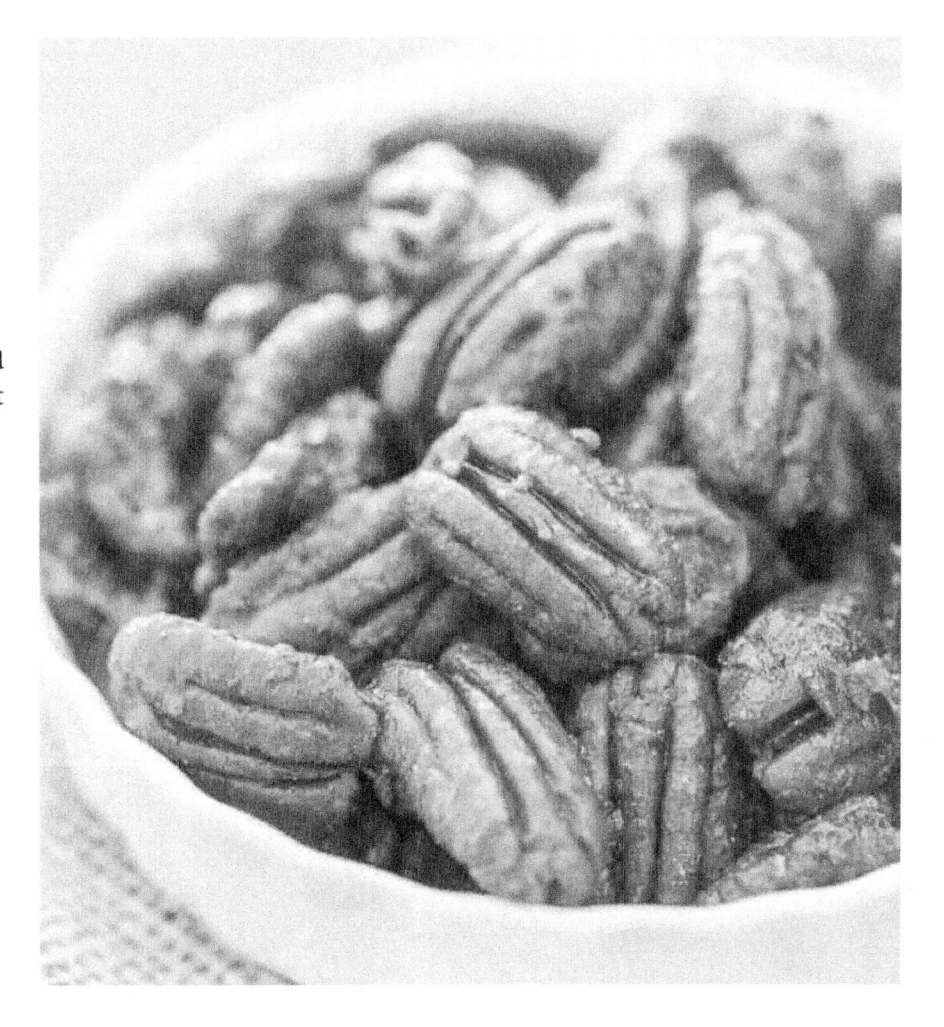

1. Preheat oven to 325°F.
2. In a small bowl combine the first 3 ingredients. Set aside.
3. In a large bowl, whisk the water with the egg white until airy and light. Add the pecan halves and stir to coat.
4. Sprinkle the sugar mixture over the pecans. Mix together evenly and spread evenly onto a parchment-lined baking sheet.
5. Bake for about 40 minutes, until pecans are browned and the sugar has caramelized. Be sure to stir the pecans regularly as they cook.

Recipe Notes:

1. Add your favorite spices like pumpkin pie spice, ginger, or apple pie spice.
2. Try a small pinch of cayenne pepper or 1 teaspoon of vanilla extra added to the egg.
3. Swap out the pecans for other nuts like cashews, almonds, or walnuts.
4. Add candied pecans to salad (especially great with kale winter salad or spinach salad).
5. Add them to a bowl of yogurt, crush them over a breakfast smoothie or smoothie bowl.
6. Drizzle with dark chocolate to take them to the next level.
7. Place them in a mason jar and tie it with a ribbon as a nice homemade gift.

NUTRITION FACTS

Serving: 0.25cup, Calories: 246, Carbohydrates: 17g, Protein: 3g, Fat: 20g, Saturated Fat: 2g, Sodium: 149mg, Potassium: 119mg, Fiber: 3g, Sugar: 14g, Vitamin A: 16IU, Vitamin C: 1mg, Calcium: 21mg, Iron: 1mg

Spritz Cookies

PREP TIME: 10 minutes
COOK TIME: 7 minutes
TOTAL TIME: 17 minutes

Serves: 40

4

Flavored with almond extract and portioned out with a cookie press, it's easy to churn out dozens of yummy cookies.

- 1 cup butter softened
- 1 ¼ cups powdered sugar
- ½ teaspoon salt
- 1 large egg
- ½ teaspoon vanilla extract
- ½ teaspoon almond extract
- 2 ½ cups flour

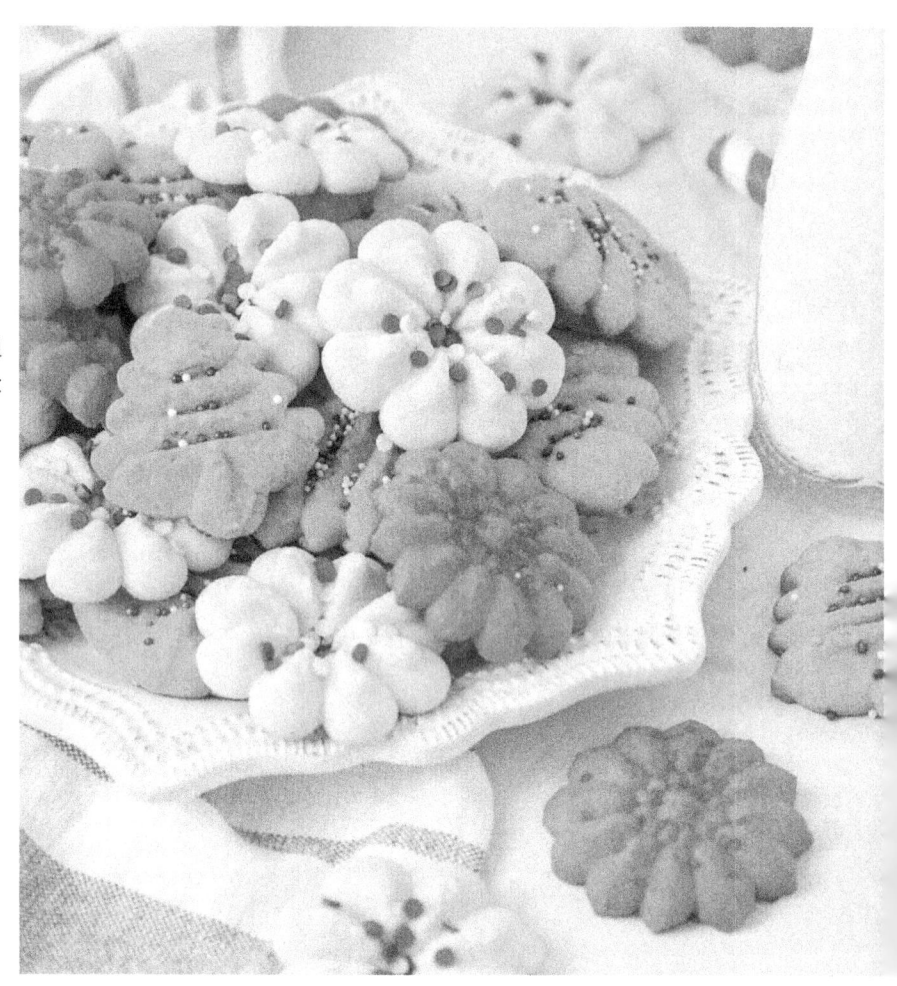

1. Preheat oven to 375°F.
2. With a mixer on medium speed, cream butter, powdered sugar, and salt until fluffy. Mix in egg, vanilla, and almond extract.
3. Add flour a little bit at a time beating after each addition.
4. Place dough into a cookie press. Squeeze cookies about 1 ½" apart and add sprinkles if desired.
5. Bake 7-9 minutes.

Recipe Notes:
1. Ensure all ingredients are room temperature.
2. Make a spice spritz by adding a teaspoon of ground cinnamon and half a teaspoon of ground nutmeg.

No Cookie Press? No problem!
1. To make spritz cookies without a cookie press, roll out the dough and use cookie cutters or a glass to cut out round shapes. Or, shape into one-inch balls and press them with anything that has a design, the bottom of a glass can leave a pretty design.

NUTRITION FACTS

Serving: 1cookie, Calories: 86, Carbohydrates: 10g, Protein: 1g, Fat: 5g, Saturated Fat: 3g, Cholesterol: 16mg, Sodium: 71mg, Potassium: 11mg, Fiber: 1g, Sugar: 4g, Vitamin A: 148IU, Calcium: 3mg, Iron: 1mg

Chocolate Peppermint Cookies

PREP TIME 15 minutes
COOK TIME 20 minutes
CHILL TIME 1 hour
TOTAL TIME 1 hour 35 minutes

Serves: 36

7

Homemade butter Cookies are dipped in chocolate and sprinkled with peppermint candy to create these delicious, festive cookies!

- 1 cup unsalted butter room temperature
- 1 cup granulated sugar
- 3 large egg yolks room temperature
- 1 teaspoon peppermint extract
- 3 cups all-purpose flour
- ½ teaspoon salt
- 2 cups dark chocolate melting wafers
- ¼ cup crushed peppermint candies

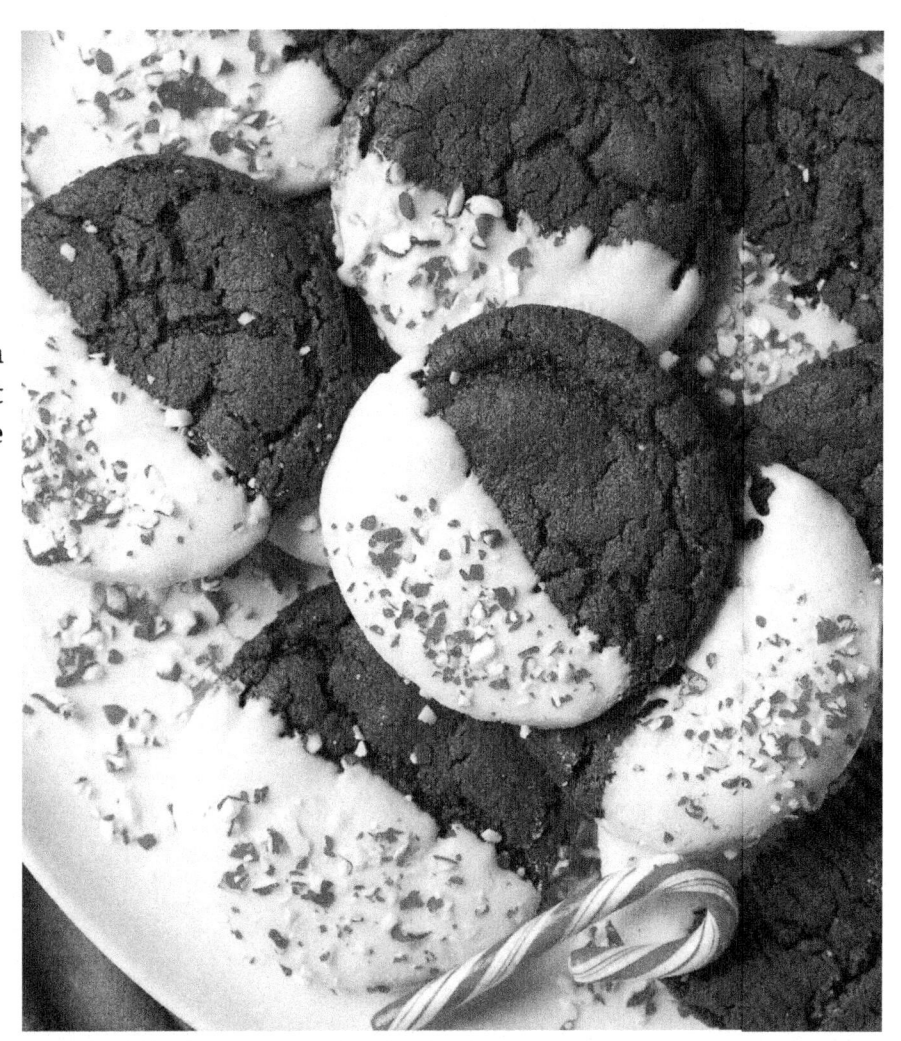

1. Cream butter and sugar in a stand mixer for 3 to 4 minutes until light and fluffy, scraping down the sides as needed. Ensure you allow the full 3-4 minutes, this step is very important.
2. Add the egg yolks and peppermint extract and mix for 30 seconds.
3. Stir in the flour a little bit at a time mixing until combined. If the dough doesn't hold together, it needs to be mixed a little bit longer.
4. Divide the dough in half and shape it into two logs, about 2" in diameter. Roll each log in parchment paper and chill for at least 1 hour (or up to 48 hours).
5. Remove from the refrigerator and preheat the oven to 375°F and line a baking sheet with parchment paper.
6. Unwrap the dough and slice into ½" thick slices. Place the doug on parchment lined pans about 1" apart.
7. Bake for 10 to 12 minutes, just until the edges start to lightly brown. Cool completely on a wire rack.
8. Melt the chocolate wafers in a bowl in the microwave on 30-second intervals stirring between each addition until fully melted.
9. Dip half of each cookie in the chocolate and place on parchment or wax paper to set.
10. Sprinkle the chocolate with crushed peppermint candy before the chocolate hardens.

NUTRITION FACTS

Calories: 167, Carbohydrates: 23g, Protein: 2g, Fat: 7g, Saturated Fat: 4g, Cholesterol: 29mg, Sodium: 125mg, Potassium: 42mg, Fiber: 1g, Sugar: 10g, Vitamin A: 180IU, Calcium: 9mg, Iron: 1mg

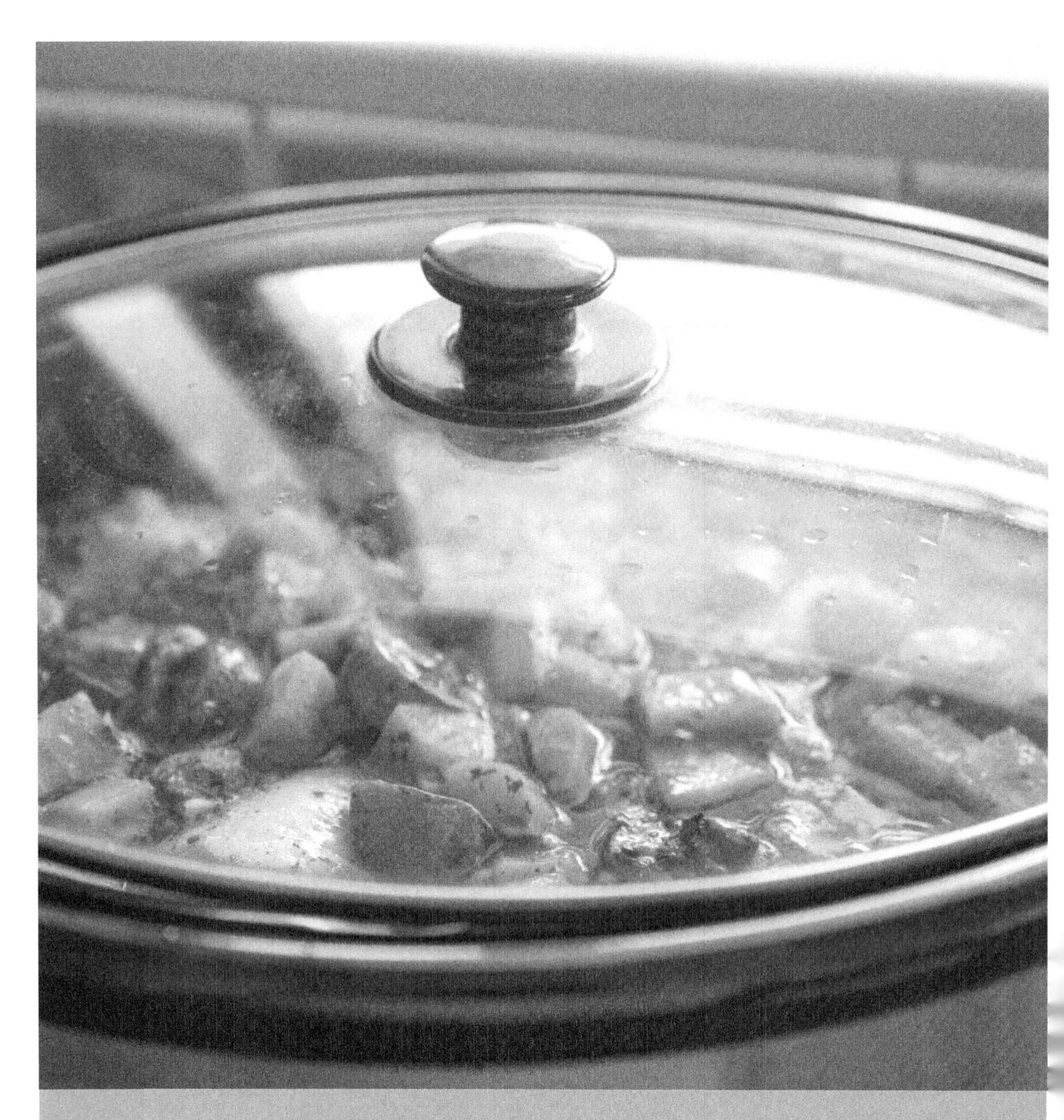

Chapter 4:
Slow Cook

CrockPot Spinach Artichoke Dip

PREP TIME: 15 minutes **Serves:** 16
COOK TIME: 1 hour
TOTAL TIME: 1 hour 15 minutes

6

Spinach Artichoke Dip is slow-cooked in the Crockpot for the ultimate creamy & cheesy appetizer!

- 12 ounces cream cheese softened, 1 ½ blocks
- 1 cup sour cream
- 2 cloves garlic minced, more to taste
- 16 oz frozen chopped spinach* thawed and squeezed dry
- 12 ounces marinated artichoke hearts chopped
- 2 cups mozzarella cheese shredded
- 1 cup parmesan cheese shredded

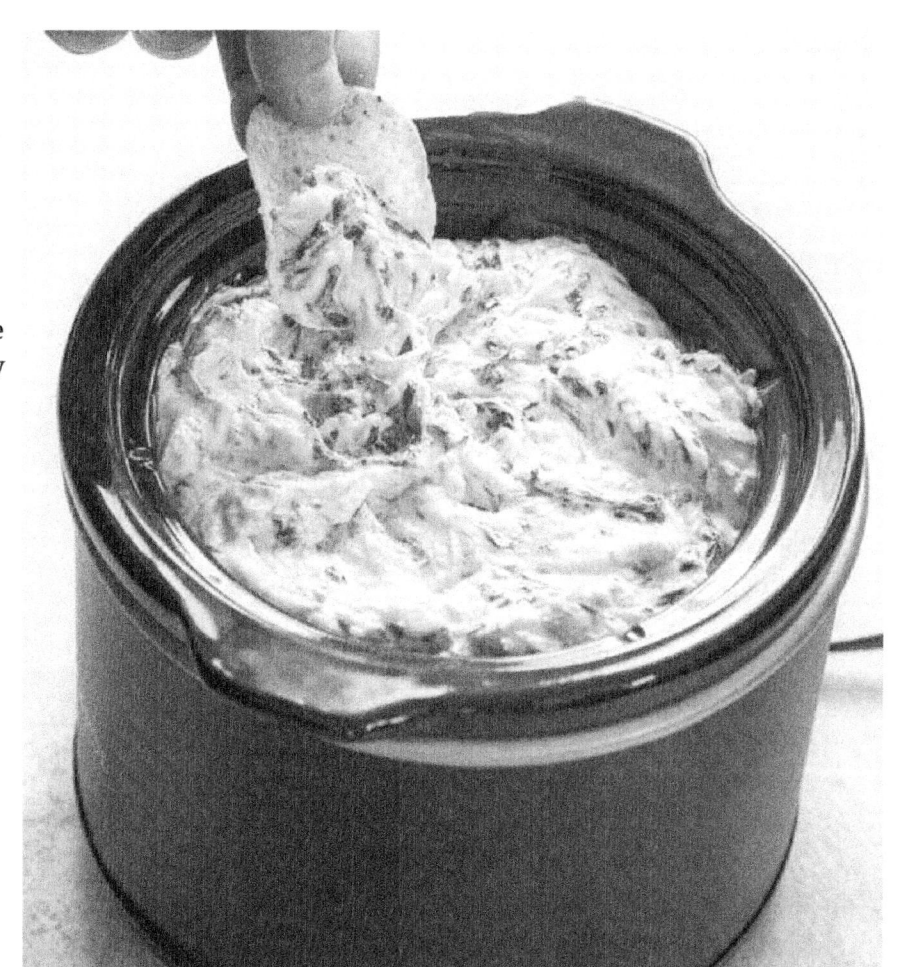

1. Combine cream cheese, sour cream, and garlic together in a large bowl and beat with a hand blender until fluffy.
2. Stir in spinach, artichokes, and cheeses, mix until fully combined. Taste and season with additional salt if desired
3. Place in a 6qt crockpot and cook on high for 1 hour or low for 2 hours. Stir and turn slow cooker to warm.

Recipe Notes:
1. This is a large recipe intended for a 6qt slow cooker. If your slow cooker is 4qt or smaller, the recipe can be halved.
2. *Spinach: Our store sells 16oz of frozen chopped spinach. If you can only find 10-12 oz packages, you can use one package.
3. Artichokes: Use marinated artichoke hearts for the best results. If your artichokes are water- packed (instead of oil), add 1/2 teaspoon Italian seasoning to the cream cheese mixture.
4. Up to 1 cup of the mozzarella can be swapped out for gruyere, swiss, or Monterey jack cheese.
5. Ensure cream cheese is at room temperature for best results. Using a hand mixer is not required but adds extra air to the cream cheese and makes it fluffy and easier to scoop.
6. Once the dip is heated through, turn the crockpot to warm. If it overheats the cheese can separate causing the dip to get oily.
7. This dip can be baked at 400°F about 20 minutes until browned and bubbly on the top.

NUTRITION FACTS

Calories: 241, Carbohydrates: 5g, Protein: 9g, Fat: 21g, Saturated Fat: 11g, Polyunsaturated Fat: 1g, Monounsaturated Fat: 5g, Cholesterol: 57mg, Sodium: 385mg, Potassium: 180mg, Fiber: 1g, Sugar: 2g, Vitamin A: 4195IU, Vitamin C: 6mg, Calcium: 235mg, Iron: 1mg

Crock Pot Pork Chops (with gravy)

PREP TIME: 15 minutes **Serves:** 4
COOK TIME: 7 hours
TOTAL TIME: 7 hours 15 minutes

6

These easy Crock Pot Pork Chops are one of our all-time favorites! Tender pork chops cooked to perfection, smothered in mushrooms and onions creating a flavorful gravy.

- 4 pork chops thick with bone-in is best, about 3 lbs
- salt & pepper to taste
- ½ teaspoon paprika
- ½ teaspoon garlic powder
- 1 tablespoon olive oil
- 10.5 oz canned cream of mushroom soup
- 10.5 oz canned cream of chicken soup
- ¾ cup beef broth I prefer low sodium
- 2 cups mushrooms sliced
- 1 small onion sliced

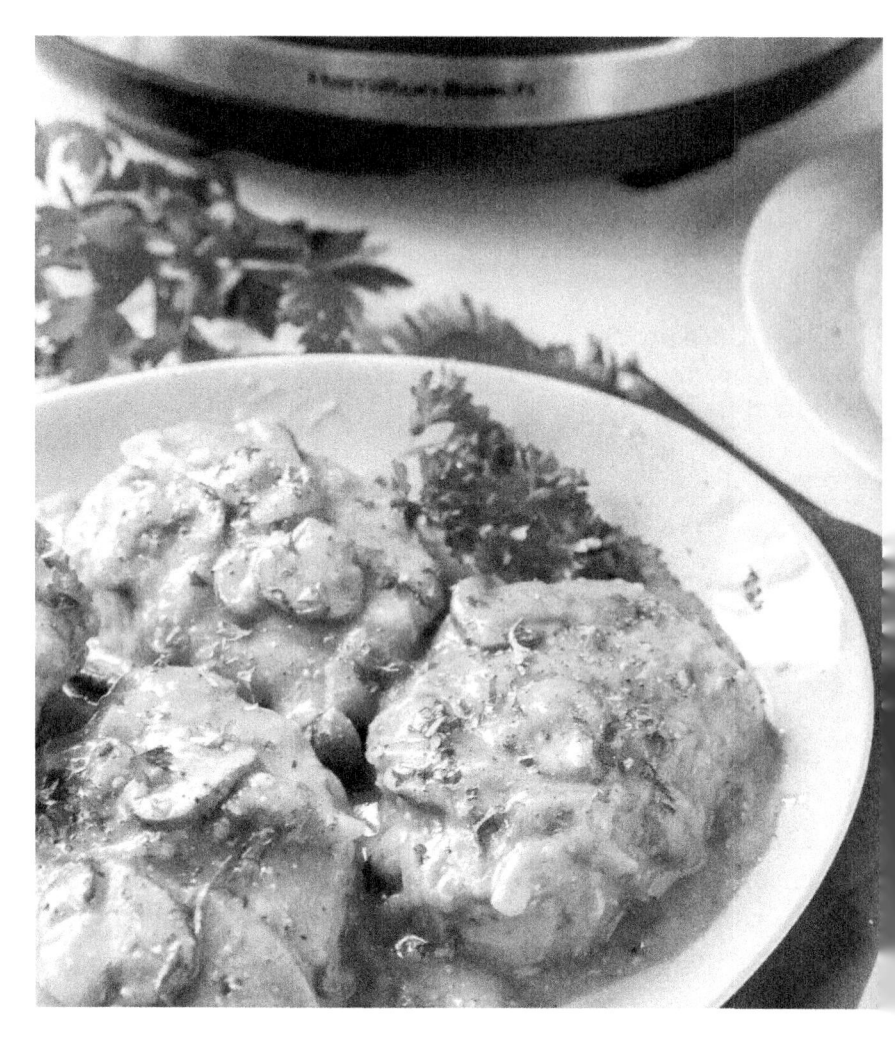

1. Preheat oil over medium-high heat. Season pork with salt, pepper, paprika and garlic powder. Brown pork on each side (about 3 minutes each side).
2. Remove pork, add soup and broth to the pan and whisk to release any brown bits in the bottom.
3. Place mushrooms and onions in the bottom of the slow cooker. Top with pork and pour the soup mixture over the top.
4. Cook on low for 7-8 hours or until pork is tender. Thicken sauce with a slurry (see notes) if desired. Serve over rice, potatoes or noodles.

Recipe Notes:

1. *The best pork chops for this recipe include blade chop, shoulder chop, sirloin chop, or tenderloin chops. Leaner cuts do work but the results are not as tender.
2. Use the canned soups directly from the can, do not add milk or water. Any type of "cream of" soup will work the combination in the recipe is our favorite.
3. If your pork chops are not tender they likely need more time.
4. To make a cornstarch slurry combine 1 tablespoon each cornstarch and water. Whisk into the sauce in the slow cooker and let it thicken for about 5 minutes.

NUTRITION FACTS

Calories: 265, Carbohydrates: 4g, Protein: 31g, Fat: 13g, Saturated Fat: 3g, Cholesterol: 89mg, Sodium: 239mg, Potassium: 716mg, Fiber: 1g, Sugar: 2g, Vitamin A: 125IU, Vitamin C: 3.1mg, Calcium: 18mg, Iron: 1.1mg

Ham and Bean Soup (Crock Pot Version)

PREP TIME: 10 minutes   **Serves:** 4
COOK TIME: 6 hours
TOTAL TIME: 6 hours 10 minutes

5

Crock Pot Ham and Bean Soup is one of our all time favorite foods to come home to on a chilly day. This "no-soaking required" Ham and Bean soup takes just minutes to prepare and cooks effortlessly in your Crock Pot all day long! Dinner is ready when you are!

- 1 package Hurst's® HamBeens® 15 Bean Soup®
- 8 cups low sodium chicken broth can sub water, beef, or vegetable broth for added flavor
- 1 leftover ham bone with meat or ham hocks, diced ham or 1 lb. cooked sausage
- 1 onion diced
- 1 clove garlic minced
- 1 teaspoon chili powder optional
- 15 ounces diced tomatoes
- 1 lemon juiced
- Optional: Hot sauce or crushed red pepper to taste

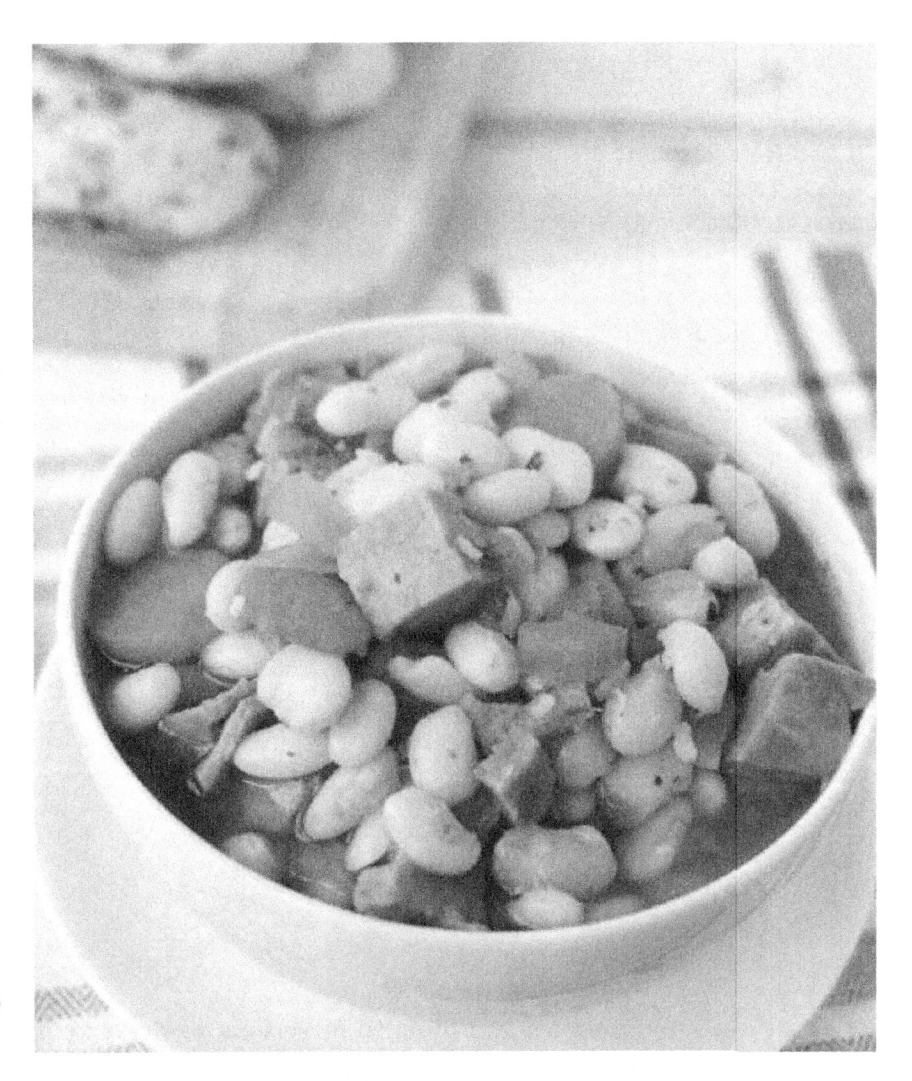

1. Rinse beans and drain. Sort any unwanted debris and set seasoning packet aside.
2. Place beans, onions, ham bone (or diced ham), broth/water, garlic and chili powder in a 6qt slow cooker.
3. Cook on high 5 hours (or low for 7-8) or until beans are tender.
4. Once tender, remove the hambone (if used) and chop any meat left on the bone and add it back to the pot.
5. Stir in diced tomatoes, Ham Flavor packet, and lemon juice.
6. Cook for additional 30 minutes.

Recipe Notes:

1. It is important that acidic ingredients are not added until the beans are soft. Check that the beans are soft before adding the diced tomatoes and lemon juice.
2. Use a leftover ham bone in this soup. If you don't have one, ask at the deli counter for ham bones (they are usually really inexpensive) or ham hocks. Leftover chopped ham works beautifully in this recipe too.
3. Rinse beans well and check for any debris. No soaking is needed when using a slow cooker. If you have already soaked the beans, you can reduce the liquid in the recipe by 1 cup.
4. For a thinner consistency, add one extra cup of broth or water to the slow cooker. For a thicker bean soup, remove a cup or so of the beans, blend them, and add them back into the soup.

NUTRITION FACTS

Calories: 259, Carbohydrates: 34g, Protein: 18g, Fat: 5g, Saturated Fat: 1g, Cholesterol: 14mg, Sodium: 387mg, Potassium: 960mg, Fiber: 8g, Sugar: 2g, Vitamin A: 95IU, Vitamin C: 12mg, Calcium: 77mg, Iron: 3.4mg

Crock Pot Mac and Cheese

PREP TIME: 15 minutes Serves: 8
COOK TIME: 2 hours
TOTAL TIME: 2 hours 15 minutes

26

Crock Pot Mac and Cheese is one of our favorite comfort food dishes! The whole family will love this creamy & cheesy dish.

- 2 cups uncooked elbow macaroni
- 10 ½ ounces condensed cream of chicken soup
- 3 cups cheddar cheese shredded
- 1 cup gruyere cheese shredded
- ½ cup mayonnaise
- ½ cup sour cream regular or light
- 1 teaspoon onion powder
- ½ teaspoon dry mustard powder
- ½ teaspoon pepper

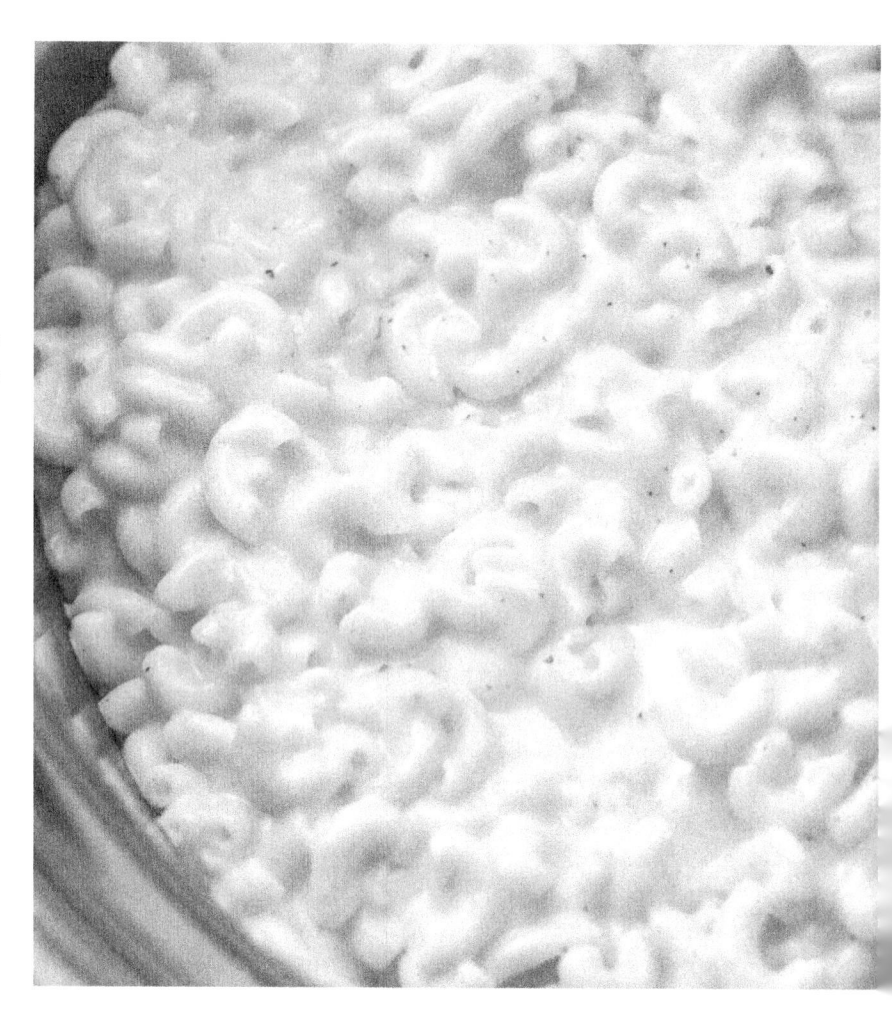

1. Boil macaroni noodles according to directions to make them very al dente. (I cook them for at least 1-2 minutes less than directed on the bag. Mine boiled for 5 minutes). Drain and rinse under cold water.
2. Combine all ingredients in a 4qt slow cooker and cook on high for 2 hours or low for 3 hours, stirring once or twice.
3. Serve hot.

Recipe Notes:

1. Pasta - Do not overcook the pasta, it should be very firm after boiling. Rinsing the pasta stops it from cooking.
2. Cheese - Shred the cheese from a block, pre-shredded cheeses do not work as well. If you do not have gruyere cheese, you can use 4 cups cheddar instead.
3. Cooking time - Check the pasta early, slow cookers can vary.
4. Double the recipe - To double this recipe, use a 6QT crockpot. Cook on high for 2 1/2 hours, stirring after 1 hour and 2 hours. (When stirring, try to do it as quickly as possible to keep the heat inside).
5. Make ahead - To prepare this ahead of time, mix all of the ingredients except the pasta. The pasta can be cooked ahead, rinsed, and cooled. Combine the pasta and sauce ingredients in the crockpot just before cooking.
6. Baking in the oven - If you prefer or if you are short on time, you can bake this in the oven (and I have many many times!) Preheat the oven to 350°F. Bake 30 minutes covered and 30 minutes uncovered.

NUTRITION FACTS

Calories: 464, Carbohydrates: 31g, Protein: 27g, Fat: 47g, Saturated Fat: 21g, Cholesterol: 105mg, Sodium: 917mg, Potassium: 203mg, Fiber: 1g, Sugar: 2g, Vitamin A: 1000IU, Vitamin C: 0.2mg, Calcium: 665mg, Iron: 1.5mg

Crockpot Meatballs

PREP TIME: 10 minutes Serves: 8
COOK TIME: 3 hours
TOTAL TIME: 3 hours 10 minutes

8

Tender juicy meatballs in an easy tomato sauce requires very little prep and has amazing flavor!

Meatballs

- 1 ½ pounds lean ground beef
- ⅓ cup Italian bread crumbs
- ¼ cup onion finely diced
- 1 teaspoon Italian seasoning
- 1 egg
- ¼ cup parsley fresh, chopped
- ¼ cup parmesan cheese

Sauce

- 24 ounces pasta sauce
- 2 cloves garlic
- 14 ounces crushed tomatoes canned
- 28 ounces diced tomatoes canned, undrained
- 1 teaspoon Italian seasoning

1. Spray slow cooker with cooking spray.
2. Combine all meatball ingredients in a bowl. Using a tablespoon, form 24 meatballs. Place uncooked meatballs in the bottom of the slow cooker.
3. Combine all sauce ingredients in a large bowl. Pour over meatballs and cook on high for 3-4 hours.
4. Serve over pasta.

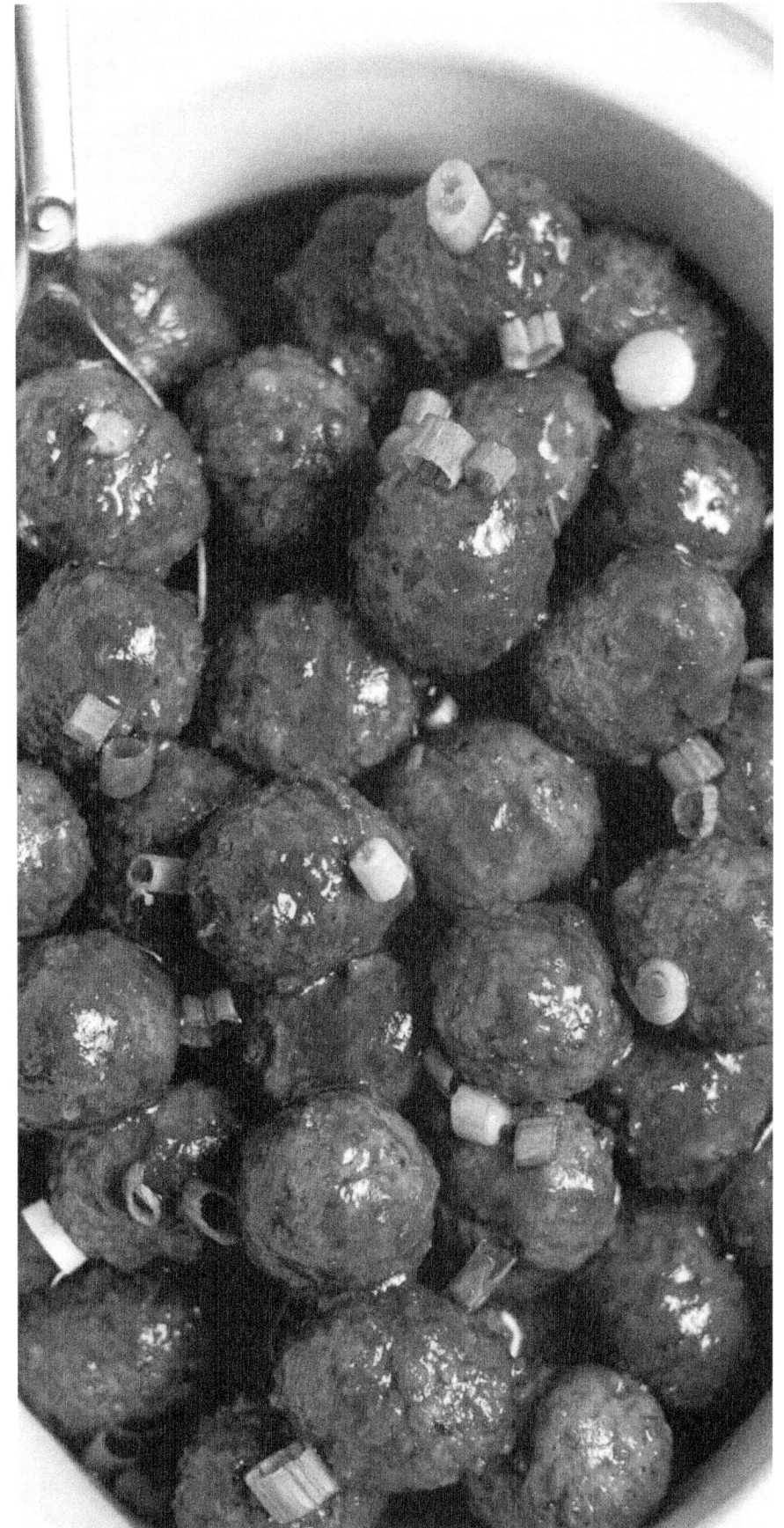

NUTRITION FACTS

Calories: 280, Carbohydrates: 16g, Protein: 21g, Fat: 14g, Saturated Fat: 5g, Cholesterol: 80mg, Sodium: 703mg, Potassium: 901mg, Fiber: 3g, Sugar: 8g, Vitamin A: 815IU, Vitamin C: 23mg, Calcium: 133mg, Iron: 4.9mg

Easy Crock Pot Chili Recipe

PREP TIME: 15 minutes   **Serves:** 10
COOK TIME: 4 hours
TOTAL TIME: 4 hours 15 minutes

5

This Easy Crockpot Chili recipe is loaded with ground beef, seasonings, & tons of flavor.

- 3 pounds lean ground beef *see note
- 2 medium onions diced, ½-inch
- 4 cloves garlic minced
- 1 can or bottle light beer approx. 12 oz
- 28 ounces whole tomatoes with juice
- 14 ounces diced tomatoes with juice
- 1 medium green bell pepper ½" diced, optional
- 14 ounces tomato sauce
- 15 ounces kidney beans drained and rinsed
- Seasoning Mixture
- 4 tablespoons chili powder
- 1 tablespoon cumin
- 2 teaspoons parsley
- 1 teaspoon smoked paprika
- 1 teaspoon each salt and pepper
- 1 teaspoon oregano

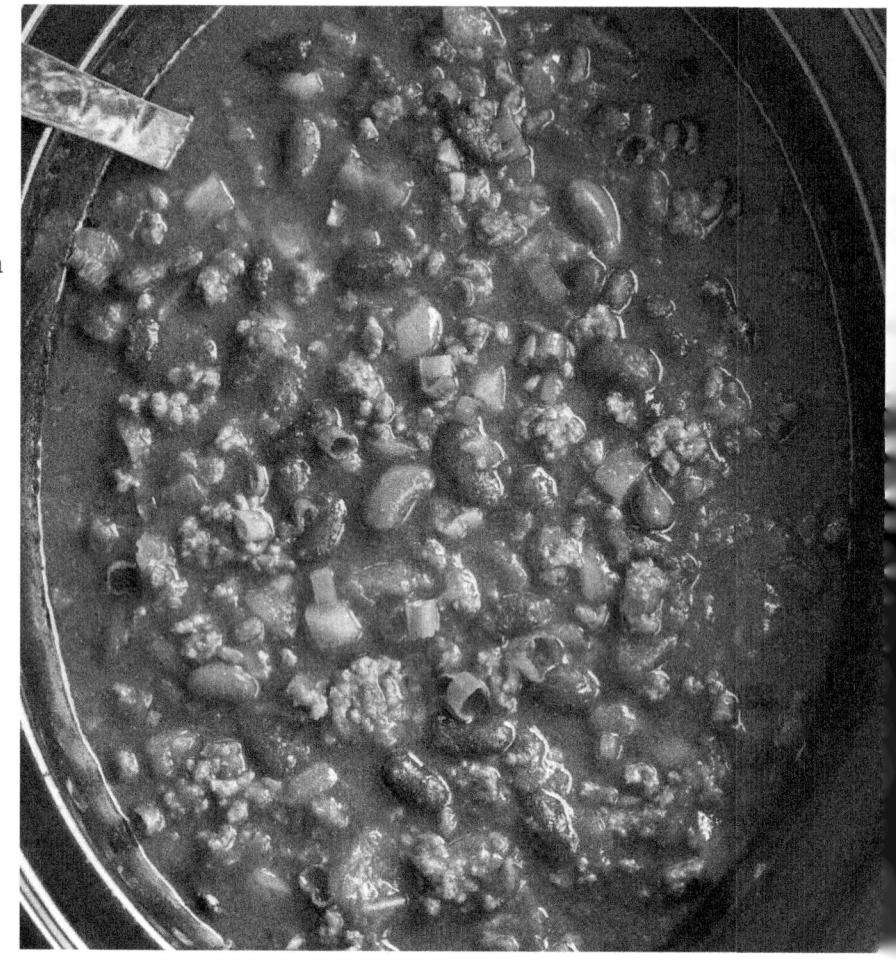

1. Combine seasoning mixture with ground beef and mix until well combined.
2. Brown ground beef*, onions, and garlic until no pink remains. Drain any fat. Add beer and simmer until most of the liquid has evaporated.
3. Combine beef mixture and all remaining ingredients in a slow cooker. If desired slightly mash the whole tomatoes.
4. Cook on high for 4 hours or low 7-8 hours. Once cooked, remove the lid and let cool slightly before serving.

Recipe Notes:

1. *This recipe can be made with 2lbs of ground beef if desired and the beans can be doubled.
2. Ground beef may need to be browned in batches depending on the size of your pan.
3. The chili will be very hot after cooking and will thicken as it cools. I allow it to cool at least 30 minutes with the lid off stirring occasionally (and it is still very hot).
4. This chili is fairly mild. Add one finely diced jalapeno or a pinch of cayenne pepper to add a little bit of heat.
5. Beer is recommended but if needed, you can skip it or substitute beef broth. I often use a light beer (such as Budweiser) but use your favorite.
6. You can add vegetables to this recipe if you'd like. Diced bell peppers, zucchini, and mushrooms are great added to crockpot chili. Veggies contain water so you might like to precook them or leave the lid off the slow cooker for the last while of cooking.
7. To thicken leave the lid off the Crockpot and let some of the liquid evaporate. Or make a slurry of equal amounts of water and corn starch in a jar. Shake the jar until the slurry is blended then slowly stir it into the chili (you might not need all of it).
8. This recipe is perfect for doubling, ensure it fits in your slow cooker (which shouldn't be more than 3/4 full). Chili freezes and reheats well.

NUTRITION FACTS

Calories: 293, Carbohydrates: 21g, Protein: 35g, Fat: 7g, Saturated Fat: 3g, Cholesterol: 84mg, Sodium: 470mg, Potassium: 1112mg, Fiber: 6g, Sugar: 5g, Vitamin A: 1365IU, Vitamin C: 16.3mg, Calcium: 93mg, Iron: 7.2mg

Crockpot Swiss Steak

PREP TIME: 20 minutes Serves: 4
COOK TIME: 6 hours 15 minutes
TOTAL TIME: 6 hours 35 minutes

6

Tender pieces of steak are slow-cooked with a rich tomato brown gravy!

- 1 ½ pounds round steak or cube steaks or minute steaks
- 2 carrots sliced into 1" pieces
- 1 stalk celery sliced into 1" pieces
- ½ onion sliced ½"
- 2 cloves garlic sliced
- ¼ cup flour
- 1 tablespoon olive oil
- ½ cup white wine
- 1 cup beef broth
- 14 oz canned diced tomatoes, with juice
- 2 tablespoons tomato paste
- 1 tablespoon Worcestershire sauce
- ½ teaspoon dried thyme leaves
- salt and pepper to taste
- corn starch for thickening optional

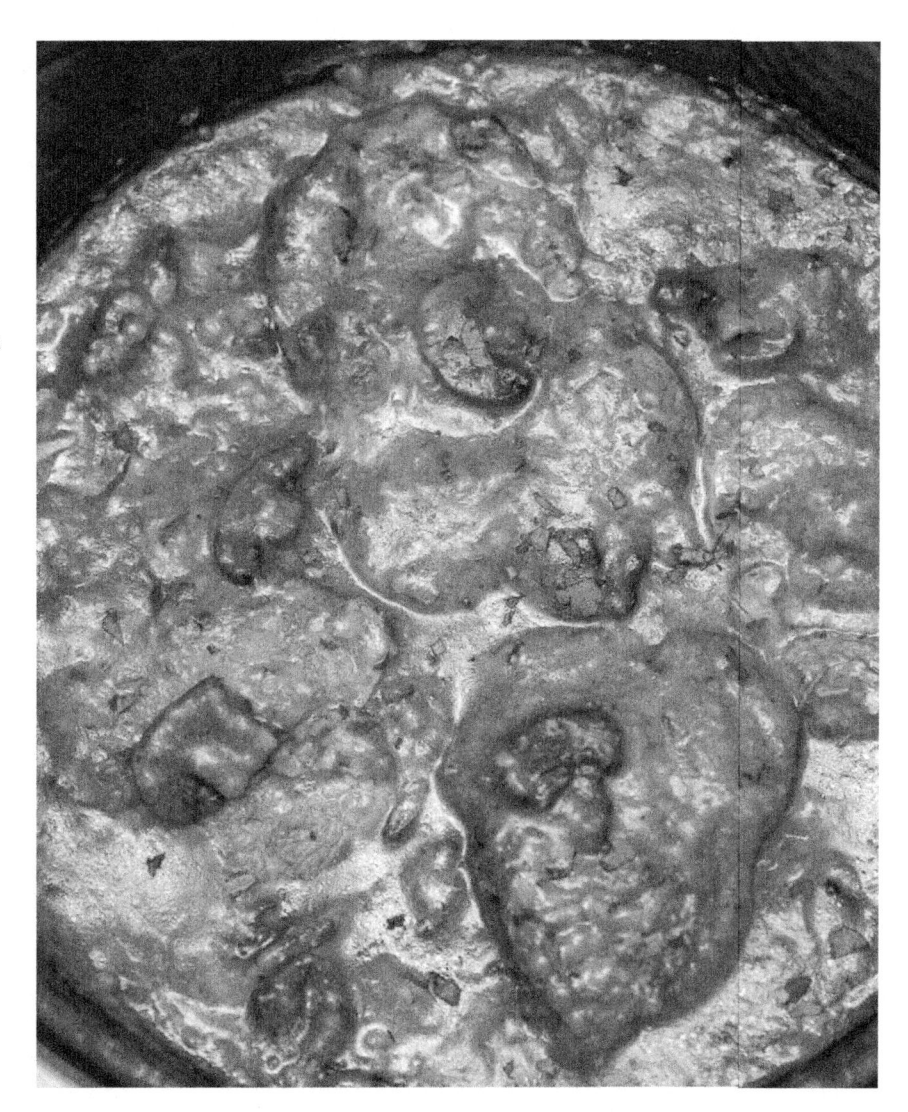

1. Add sliced carrots, celery, onion, & garlic to the bottom of a slow cooker.
2. Pound steaks with a meat tenderizer to ¼ inch thickness and season with salt and pepper (cube steaks do not need to be pounded). Put flour in a shallow dish or plate and dredge each steak in the flour mixture.
3. Heat oil in a skillet over medium-high heat and brown steaks on both sides, about 2 minutes per side adding more oil if needed.
4. In the same pan, add wine and scrape up any brown bits. Add to the slow cooker with remaining ingredients except for the cornstarch.
5. Cover and cook for 6-8 hours on low or 4-5 hours on high or until steaks are fork tender.
6. Serve over mashed potatoes or noodles.

Recipe Notes:
1. For a smoother sauce, swap out the diced tomatoes for crushed tomatoes or even canned tomato soup.
2. For extra sauce, an additional can of tomatoes can be added.
3. Optional: To thicken the sauce, combine 1 tablespoon cornstarch with 1 tablespoon water. Bring the sauce to a simmer on the stove and add a little at a time to thicken.

NUTRITION FACTS

Calories: 281, Carbohydrates: 15g, Protein: 29g, Fat: 9g, Saturated Fat: 2g, Polyunsaturated Fat: 1g, Monounsaturated Fat: 5g, Cholesterol: 71mg, Sodium: 308mg, Potassium: 838mg, Fiber: 2g, Sugar: 5g, Vitamin A: 5414IU, Vitamin C: 8mg, Calcium: 54mg, Iron: 4mg

Crock Pot Sausage Pasta

PREP TIME: 20 minutes   Serves: 6
COOK TIME: 4 hours
TOTAL TIME: 4 hours 20 minutes

12

Crock Pot sausage pasta is a set-it-and-forget-it dish loaded with veggies, sausage, & cheesy pasta!

- 1 pound Italian sausage links
- 1 onion sliced
- 1 eggplant ½" cubes, 4-5 cups
- 8 ounces mushrooms thickly sliced
- 14 ounces crushed tomatoes 1 can
- 14 ounces whole tomatoes lightly drained, 1 can
- 2 cloves garlic minced
- 1 tablespoon balsamic vinegar
- 1 teaspoon Italian seasoning
- ¼ teaspoon chili flakes
- 8 ounces medium pasta such as penne or rotini
- parmesan and fresh basil & parsley for serving

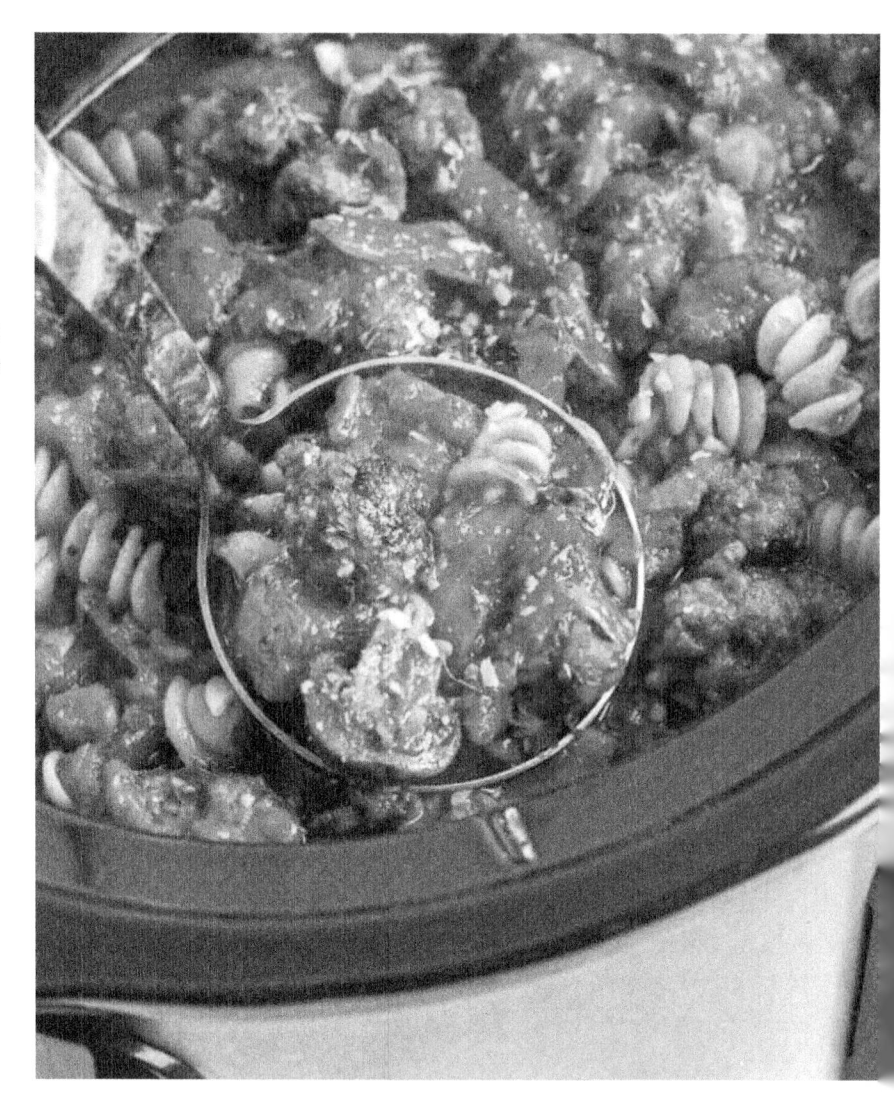

1. Remove casings from sausage and break into large pieces. Brown in a skillet over medium heat making sure that you don't break the meat up too much. Drain fat.
2. Place onion, eggplant, sausage, and mushrooms into the bottom of a 6qt slow cooker. Top with Sausage.
3. Combine crushed and whole tomatoes (slightly squished), garlic, vinegar, & seasonings. Pour over the sausage and vegetables.
4. Cover and cook on low 7-8 hours or high for 4 hours.
5. Before serving, cook pasta according to package directions. Once cooked, stir pasta into the sauce.
6. Top with parmesan cheese and fresh herbs for serving.

Recipe Notes:
1. Eggplant can be substituted with other vegetables like bell peppers or zucchini. If using, zucchini should be added during the last hour of cooking so it doesn't get mushy.
2. Cook pasta to al dente (firm) so it doesn't overcook when added to the other ingredients.
3. Sausage can be replaced with ground beef or turkey, you will need to add extra Italian seasoning and a 1/2 teaspoon fennel seeds if you have it. Chili flakes can be added.

NUTRITION FACTS

Serving: 1.5cups, Calories: 355, Carbohydrates: 34g, Protein: 15g, Fat: 19g, Saturated Fat: 7g, Cholesterol: 43mg, Sodium: 557mg, Potassium: 696mg, Fiber: 5g, Sugar: 8g, Vitamin A: 201IU, Vitamin C: 13mg, Calcium: 64mg, Iron: 3mg

Crockpot Split Pea Soup

PREP TIME: 15 minutes   **Serves:** 12
COOK TIME: 5 hours
TOTAL TIME: 5 hours 15 minutes

4

Warm and satisfying Crockpot Split Pea Soup is a "set it and forget it" recipe that's comforting to come home to. Healthy ingredients and easy prep make this soup a winner!

- 20 ounces dried split peas green or yellow, *see note
- 5 cups chicken broth
- 2 cups water *see note
- 1 meaty ham bone or 2 cups leftover ham
- 3 stalks celery diced
- 2 large carrots diced
- 1 large onion diced
- 2 cloves garlic minced
- 1 bay leaf
- ½ teaspoon black pepper
- ½ teaspoon thyme leaves
- 1 tablespoon fresh parsley

1. Rinse peas and drain well.
2. Combine all ingredients except parsley in a 6qt slow cooker.
3. Cover and cook on high for 4-5 hours or on low 8 hours.
4. Discard bay leaf. Stir in parsley and season with salt and pepper to taste.

Recipe Notes:

1. I use Hurst HamPeas Split Peas in this recipe which comes in a 20 oz package. If using a different brand, check the package size. If it contains only 16 oz (1 pound), do not add the additional 2 cups of water.
2. Reduce the liquid slightly for a thicker soup.
3. If cooking for 4 hours on high in the Crockpot, soak peas overnight in clean water. Drain & rinse before using.
4. No need to soak the green peas if they are slow cooking for more than 4 hours!
5. For best results, keep the bone or ham hock in until the soup is finished.
6. The peas will break down and naturally thicken the soup.
7. Thin split pea soup by stirring in extra chicken broth, and to thicken it allow it to cook with the lid off for about 1 hour.

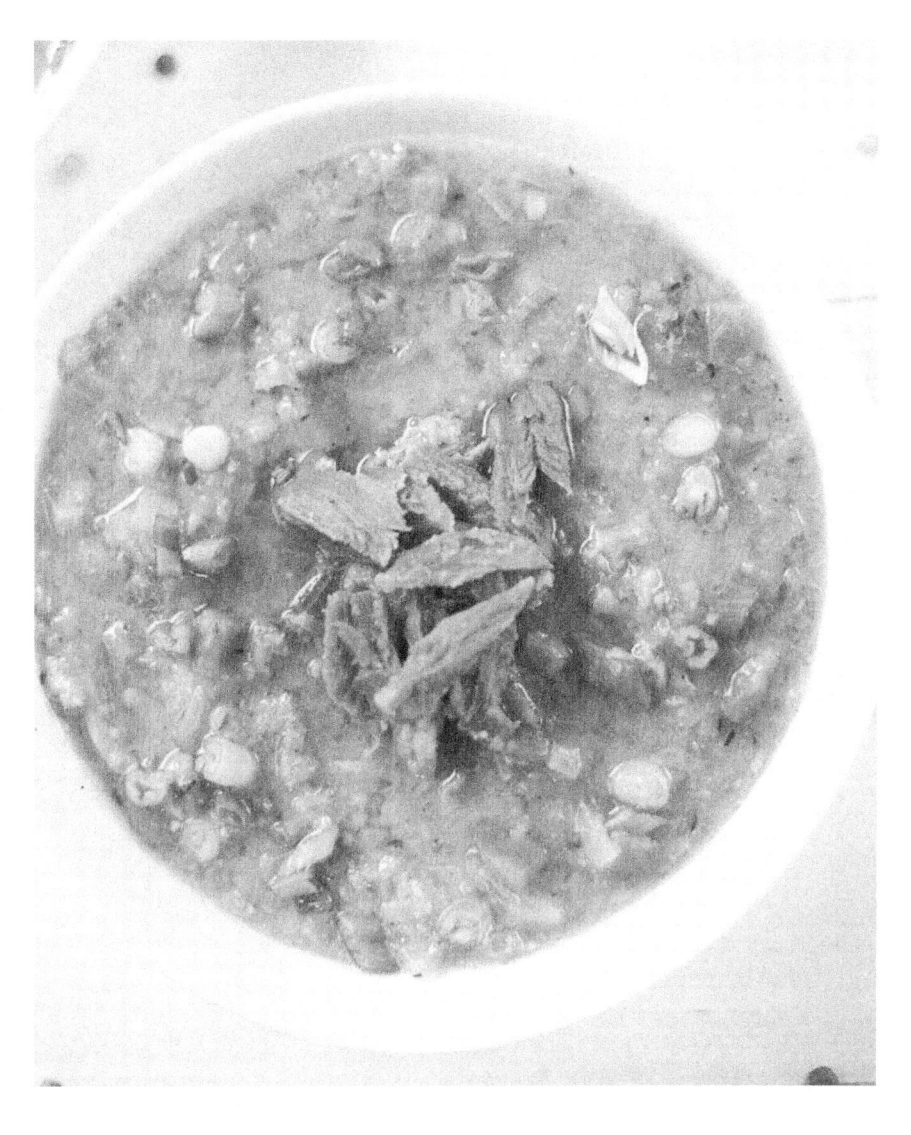

NUTRITION FACTS

Calories: 203, Carbohydrates: 26g, Protein: 15g, Fat: 5g, Saturated Fat: 2g, Cholesterol: 14mg, Sodium: 660mg, Potassium: 604mg, Fiber: 10g, Sugar: 4g, Vitamin A: 2141IU, Vitamin C: 10mg, Calcium: 42mg, Iron: 2mg

CrockPot Lasagna

PREP TIME 30 minutes
COOK TIME 3 hours 30 minutes
RESTING TIME 30 minutes
TOTAL TIME 4 hours 30 minutes

Serves: 8

22

Crockpot Lasagna is an easy set-it-and-forget-it meal that tastes just like the oven version. Layers of lasagna noodles, meat sauce, & loads of gooey cheese make an unforgettable Italian favorite in the slow cooker!

- 9 lasagna noodles uncooked
- 2 cups mozzarella cheese shredded
- ½ cup parmesan cheese grated

Sauce
- 1 pound lean ground beef
- 1 small onion diced
- 4 cloves garlic minced
- 15 ounces petite diced tomatoes
- 36 ounces marinara sauce
- 1 teaspoon Italian seasoning

Cheese Filling
- 24 oz ricotta cheese or cottage cheese
- 1 cup mozzarella cheese shredded
- ¼ cup parmesan cheese grated
- 1 egg

1. Cook ground beef, onion, and garlic in a large saucepan until no pink remains. Drain fat.
2. Stir in sauce, diced tomatoes with juices and seasoning. Simmer 5-7 minutes or until thickened. Season with salt & pepper to taste.
3. Meanwhile, mix cheese filling ingredients.
4. Spread 1 ½ cups sauce in the bottom of a 6 qt slow cooker. Top with a layer of uncooked lasagna noodles (break them to fit in the slow cooker as needed).
5. Create layers of cheese mixture, sauce, and noodles. End with pasta sauce and finally top with remaining mozzarella and parmesan.
6. Cover and cook on low for 3 to 3.5 hours or until pasta is cooked through (the edges will be brown and crispy). Turn the slow cooker off, open lid slightly to allow steam to escape and let rest 30 minutes to set.

Recipe Notes:

1. Layering order (you may or may not be able to fit 3 whole noodles on each layer depending on the shape of your slow cooker):
   1. 1.5 cups of sauce - 2 ½ to 3 noodles - 1/3 of cheese mixture
   2. 1.5 cups of sauce - 2 ½ to 3 noodles - 1/3 of cheese mixture
   3. 1.5 cups of sauce - 2 ½ to 3 noodles - 1/3 of cheese mixture
   4. remaining sauce - mozzarella

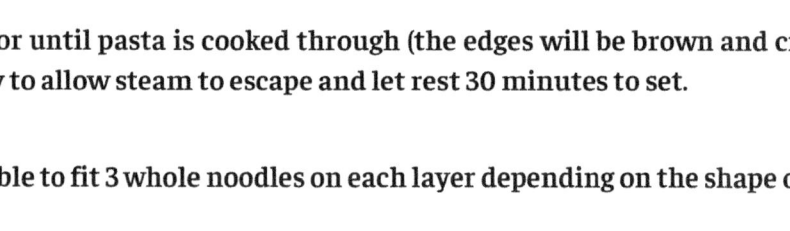

NUTRITION FACTS

Calories: 611, Carbohydrates: 40g, Protein: 40g, Fat: 33g, Saturated Fat: 18g, Trans Fat: 1g, Cholesterol: 142mg, Sodium: 1271mg, Potassium: 975mg, Fiber: 4g, Sugar: 10g, Vitamin A: 1437IU, Vitamin C: 15mg, Calcium: 561mg, Iron: 4mg

Chapter 5:
Air Fryer

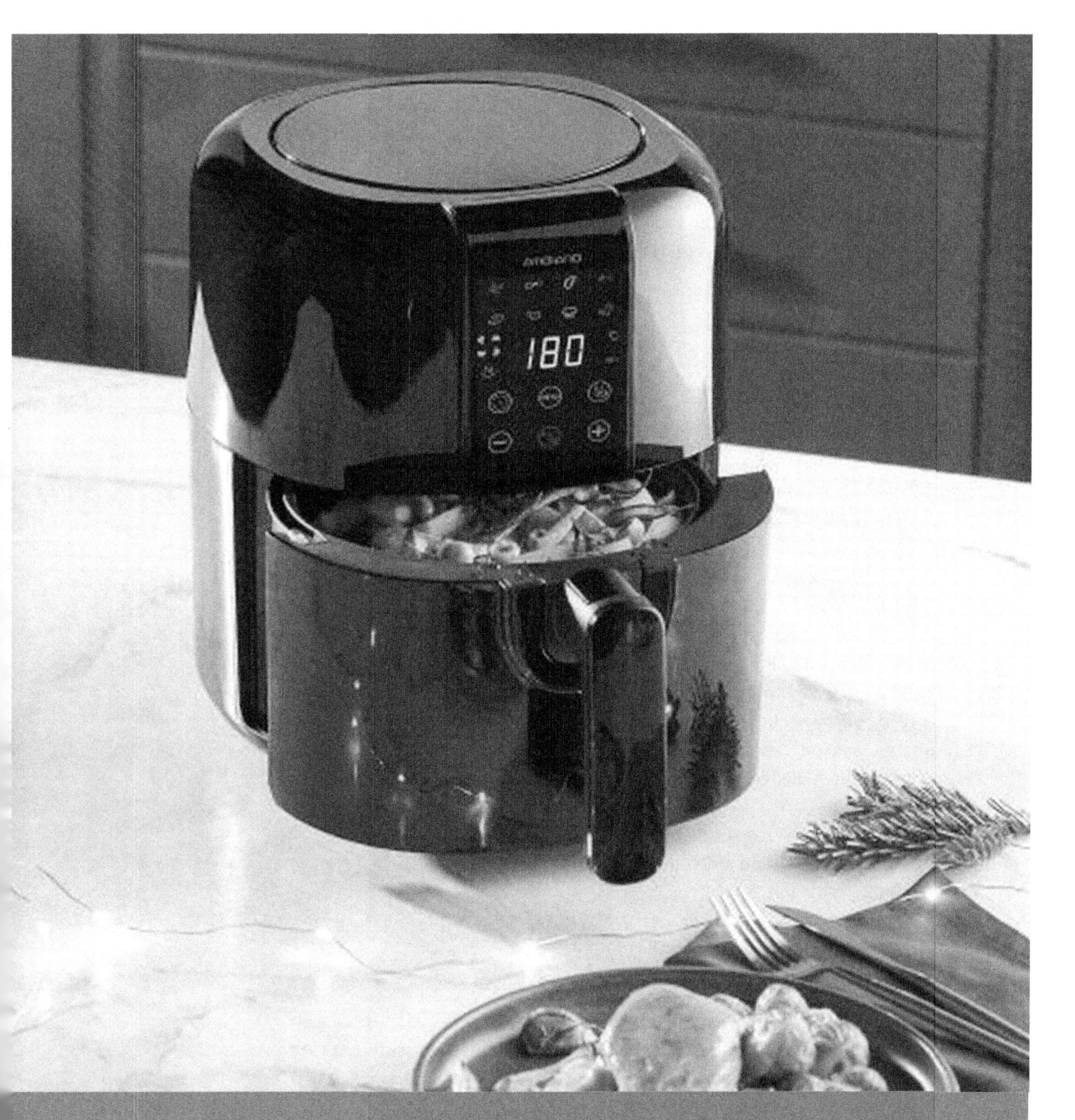

Air Fryer Chicken Legs

PREP TIME: 5 minutes
COOK TIME: 30 minutes
TOTAL TIME: 35 minutes
Serves: 4

8

These air fryer chicken legs are tender & juicy on the inside, seasoned & crispy on the outside!

- 3-4 chicken legs
- 1 tablespoon olive oil
- 1 tablespoon chicken seasoning* see note
- ½ teaspoon garlic powder
- salt & pepper to taste

1. Preheat air fryer to 370°F.
2. Pat chicken dry with a paper towel. Drizzle olive oil over chicken legs and generously season with chicken seasoning, garlic powder, and salt & pepper to taste.
3. Place the chicken legs in a single layer in the air fryer basket, skin side down, and cook for 20 minutes.
4. Flip the legs over and cook an additional 5-10 minutes or until the legs reach 165°F.

Recipe Notes:
1. *Premade chicken seasonings can vary in flavor and salt level. Season to taste or preference.
2. Homemade Chicken Seasoning
3. 1 teaspoon paprika
4. 1/2 teaspoon garlic powder
5. 1/2 teaspoon kosher salt, more or less to taste
6. 1/4 teaspoon black pepper
7. 1/4 teaspoon dried thyme leaves
8. Ensure legs aren't too crowded so air can circulate around them. Do not overlap.

NUTRITION FACTS

Calories: 242, Carbohydrates: 1g, Protein: 16g, Fat: 19g, Saturated Fat: 5g, Trans Fat: 1g, Cholesterol: 90mg, Sodium: 82mg, Potassium: 207mg, Fiber: 1g, Sugar: 1g, Vitamin A: 115IU, Vitamin C: 1mg, Calcium: 19mg, Iron: 1mg

Air Fryer Potato and Sausage

PREP TIME: 20 minutes   Serves: 4
COOK TIME: 20 minutes
TOTAL TIME: 40 minutes

15

Veggies & sausage are seasoned & air-fried until perfectly tender in this easy & flavorful recipe.

- 1 pound potatoes peeled and cut into 1" pieces
- ¾ pound smoked sausage cut in ½" slices
- 1 bell pepper diced, red or green
- ½ red onion cut in ½" pieces
- ½ cup grape tomatoes
- 1 tablespoon feta cheese optional

Seasoning

- 2 tablespoons olive oil
- 2 cloves garlic minced
- 1 teaspoon lemon juice
- ½ teaspoon dried oregano
- ½ teaspoon salt or to taste
- ¼ teaspoon black pepper
- 1 teaspoon lemon zest

1. Preheat the air fryer to 400°F.
2. Combine the seasoning ingredients in a small bowl, set aside.
3. Toss potatoes with half of the seasoning mix. Add to the air fryer basket and cook 12 minutes.
4. Toss the sausage, onion, and bell pepper with the remaining seasoning mix. Open the air fryer and shake the basket. Add the sausage and peppers and cook for 5 minutes.
5. Sprinkle with the tomatoes and feta cheese, cook 3 minutes more.

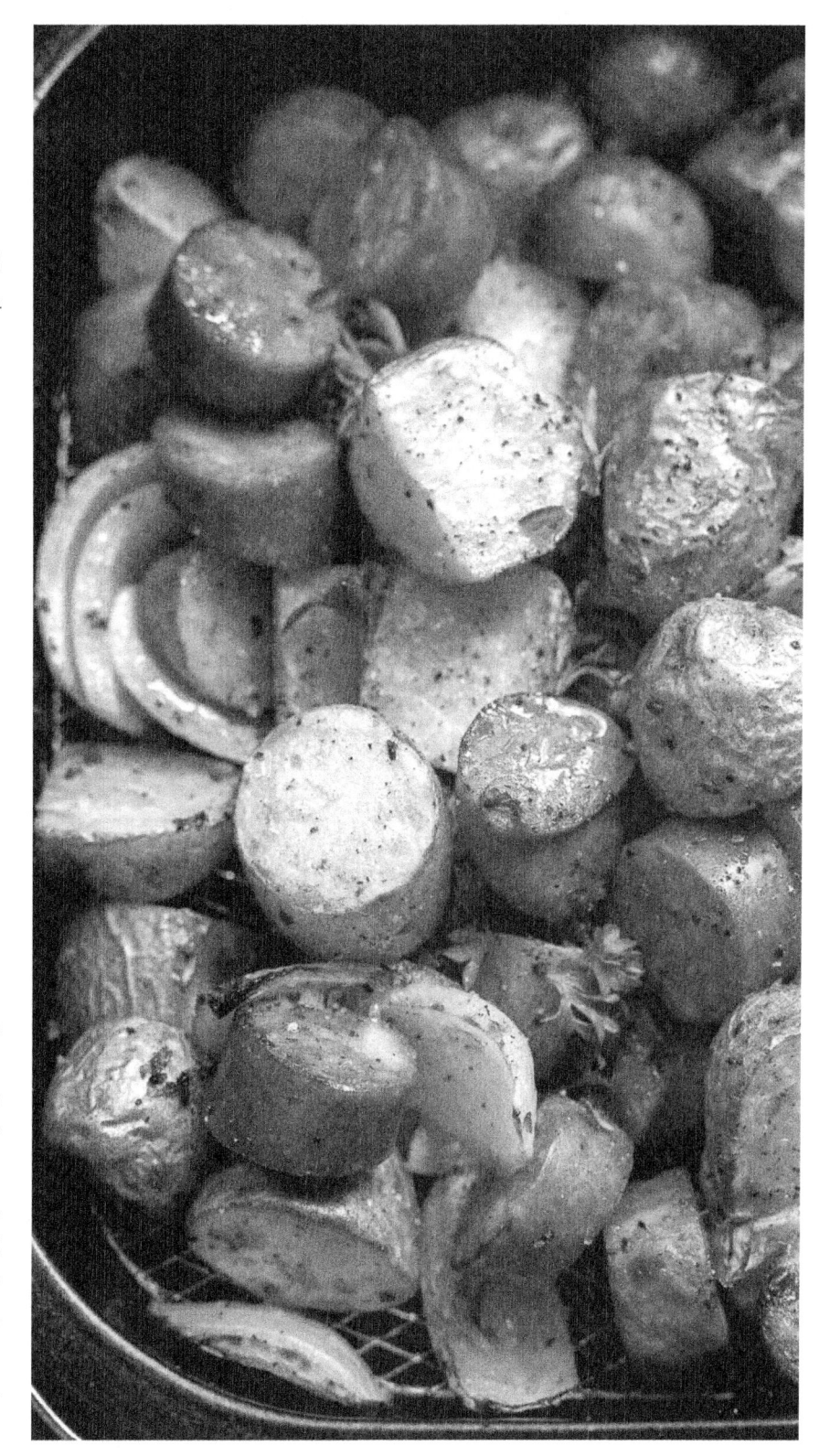

Recipe Notes:
1. Leftover sausage and potatoes can be covered in the fridge for up to 5 days. Reheat on the stovetop or in the microwave, as desired.

NUTRITION FACTS

Calories: 439, Carbohydrates: 27g, Protein: 14g, Fat: 31g, Saturated Fat: 9g, Polyunsaturated Fat: 3g, Monounsaturated Fat: 16g, Cholesterol: 64mg, Sodium: 1069mg, Potassium: 775mg, Fiber: 3g, Sugar: 3g, Vitamin A: 1111IU, Vitamin C: 49mg, Calcium: 56mg, Iron: 2mg

Air Fryer Spaghetti Squash

PREP TIME: 5 minutes
COOK TIME: 35 minutes
TOTAL TIME: 40 minutes
Serves: 4

3

Air-fryer spaghetti squash is such an easy & savory side dish that pairs perfectly with any entrèe!

- 1 medium spaghetti squash about 3 pounds
- 1 tablespoon olive oil
- ½ teaspoon kosher salt
- ¼ teaspoon black pepper

1. Preheat the air fryer to 370°F.
2. Cut the spaghetti squash in half lengthwise. Scoop out the seeds and discard (or save for roasting).
3. Brush the cut side of the squash with oil and season with salt & pepper.
4. Place cut side up in the air fryer and cook 25-30 minutes or until tender and the strands separate easily with a fork.
5. Once cooked, run a fork along the strands of the squash to separate.
6. Toss with butter if desired or season with additional salt and pepper.

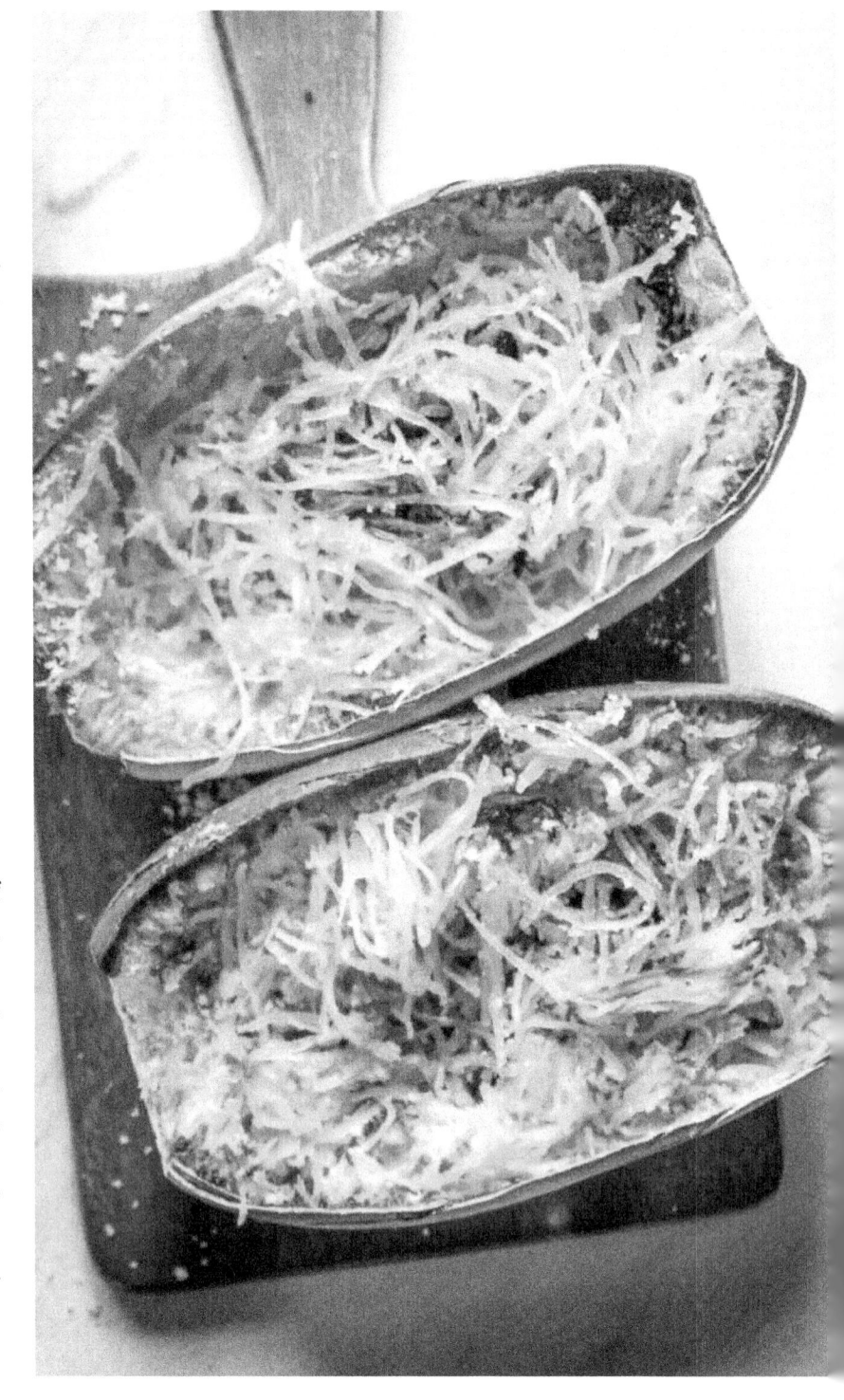

Recipe Notes:
1. Spaghetti squash seeds can be saved and cooked like pumpkin seeds.
2. Cook time can vary slightly based on the size of the squash.
3. Once the strands are separated, they can be topped with your favorite meat sauce and placed back into the squash shells. Top them with mozzarella cheese and air fryer until browned and bubbly.
4. Keep leftovers in the fridge for up to 3 days. Freeze leftovers in zippered bags for up to 6 months. Let thaw at room temperature before using.

NUTRITION FACTS

Calories: 106, Carbohydrates: 17g, Protein: 2g, Fat: 5g, Saturated Fat: 1g, Polyunsaturated Fat: 1g, Monounsaturated Fat: 3g, Sodium: 332mg, Potassium: 262mg, Fiber: 4g, Sugar: 7g, Vitamin A: 290IU, Vitamin C: 5mg, Calcium: 56mg, Iron: 1mg

Air Fryer Stuffed Chicken Breasts

PREP TIME: 15 minutes Serves: 4
COOK TIME: 25 minutes
TOTAL TIME: 40 minutes

8

Stuffed with a cream cheese mixture & air-fried until golden, these stuffed chicken breasts are a family favorite!

- 4 boneless skinless chicken breasts 5-6 ounces each
- 1 tablespoon olive oil
- ½ teaspoon paprika
- ¼ teaspoon garlic powder
- ¼ teaspoon each salt & pepper

Filling

- 3 ounces cream cheese softened
- 2 ounces feta cheese crumbled
- 1 clove garlic minced
- 1 ½ cups fresh spinach finely chopped
- 3 tablespoons red bell pepper finely diced, or tomato
- ¼ teaspoon dried oregano

1. Mix all filling ingredients in a bowl.
2. Place chicken on a cutting board and butterfly each chicken breast ¾ of the way through, do not cut all of the way through.
3. Divide filling over the chicken breasts and secure with a toothpick.
4. Preheat the air fryer to 360°F.
5. Rub the outside of the chicken with olive oil and season with paprika, garlic powder, salt & pepper.
6. Place in a single layer in the air fryer and cook 18-22 minutes or until the chicken reaches 165°F with an instant-read thermometer.

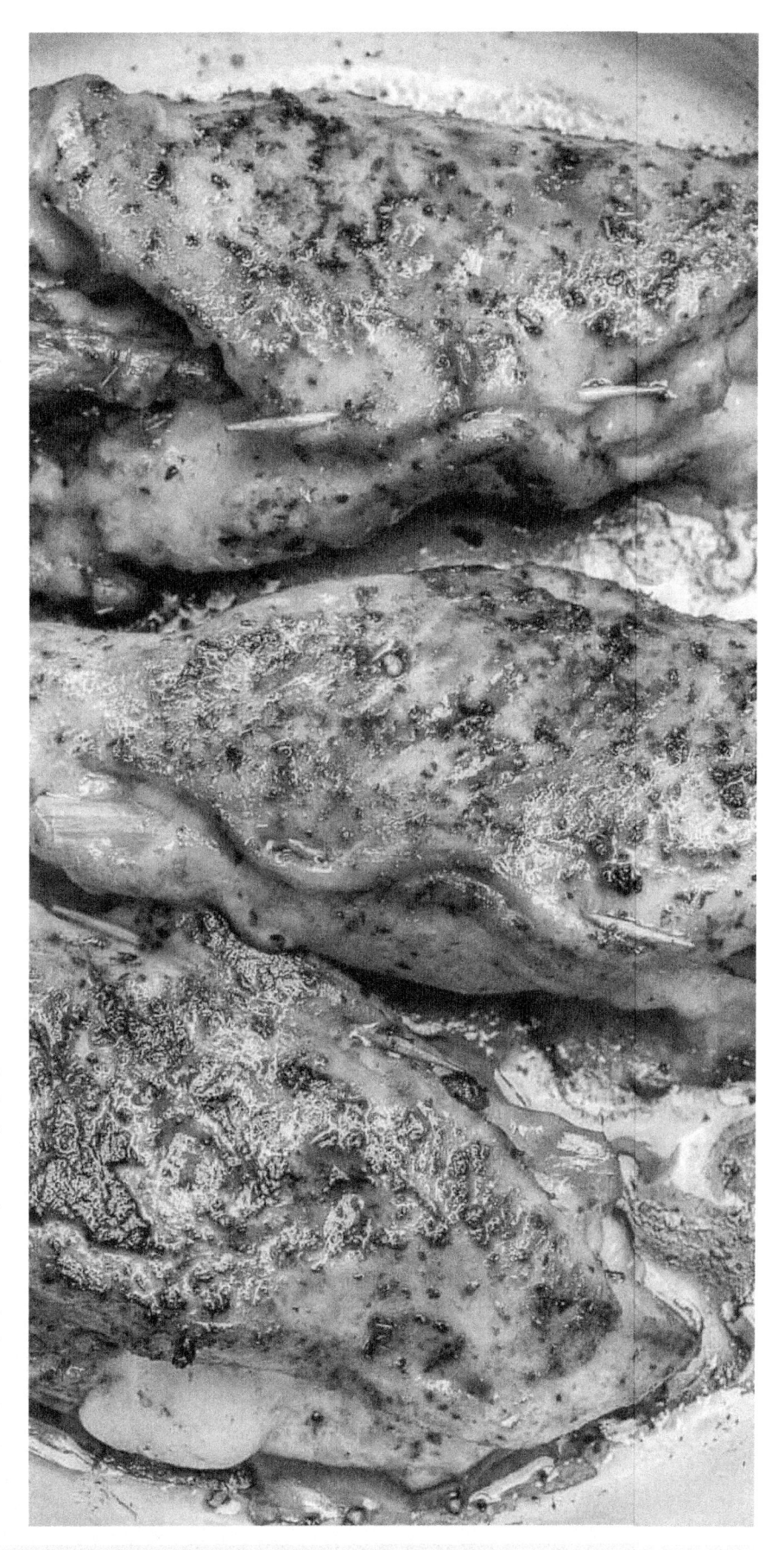

NUTRITION FACTS

Calories: 274, Carbohydrates: 2g, Protein: 28g, Fat: 17g, Saturated Fat: 7g, Polyunsaturated Fat: 1g, Monounsaturated Fat: 6g, Trans Fat: 1g, Cholesterol: 108mg, Sodium: 509mg, Potassium: 511mg, Fiber: 1g, Sugar: 1g, Vitamin A: 1208IU, Vitamin C: 4mg, Calcium: 108mg, Iron: 1mg

Lemon Pepper Wings

PREP TIME: 20 minutes Serves: 4
COOK TIME: 40 minutes
CHILL TIME: 15 minutes
TOTAL TIME: 1 hour 15 minutes

12

Lemon Pepper Wings are crispy, juicy, and perfectly seasoned!

- 1 ½ pounds chicken wings
- 1 tablespoon olive oil
- 2 teaspoons lemon pepper *see note
- 1 ½ teaspoons lemon zest
- 1 clove garlic minced, or half teaspoon garlic powder
- fresh black pepper and kosher salt
- fresh thyme and parsley for garnish optional
- 3 tablespoons melted butter
- 1 teaspoon fresh lemon juice

For Oven Method Only
- 1 teaspoon baking powder
- 1 tablespoon flour

1. Pat chicken wings dry with paper towels.

Oven Instructions
1. Preheat oven to 425°F.
2. Toss wings with flour and baking powder. Refrigerate at least 15 minutes.
3. Toss wings with olive oil, lemon pepper, lemon zest, and garlic.
4. Line a pan with foil and top with a baking rack. Spray the rack with cooking spray.
5. Bake wings 20 minutes, flip and bake an additional 15 minutes or until crisp. Broil 1 minute each side if desired.
6. Combine butter and lemon juice and toss with wings. Generously season with extra pepper, salt to taste, and fresh thyme if desired. Serve immediately.

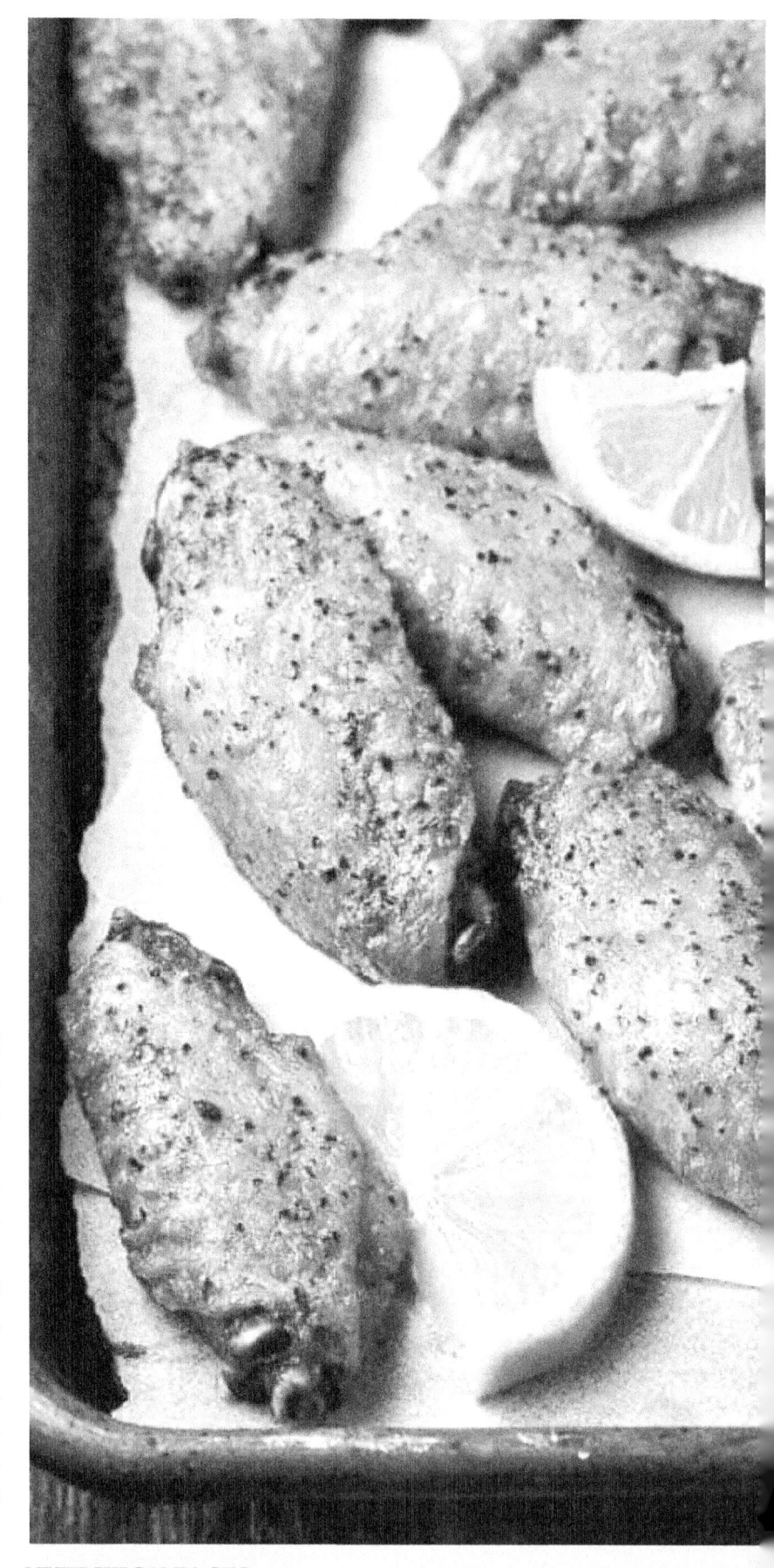

NUTRITION FACTS

Calories: 322, Carbohydrates: 3g, Protein: 17g, Fat: 27g, Saturated Fat: 10g, Trans Fat: 1g, Cholesterol: 93mg, Sodium: 143mg, Potassium: 266mg, Fiber: 1g, Sugar: 1g, Vitamin A: 403IU, Vitamin C: 1mg, Calcium: 63mg, Iron: 1mg

Air Fryer Roasted Garlic

PREP TIME: 5 minutes **Serves:** 3
COOK TIME: 30 minutes
TOTAL TIME: 35 minutes

3

Air Fryer Roasted Garlic turns out creamy & perfectly caramelized every time!

- 3 bulbs garlic
- 2 tablespoons olive oil

1. Preheat the air fryer to 380°F.
2. Cut the top ¼ of the garlic off so the cloves are exposed and drizzle with olive oil.
3. Wrap the garlic in foil and place in the air fryer basket.
4. Cook the garlic for 30-35 minutes or until it is tender and golden.
5. Remove the bulbs and gently squeeze each clove to remove it from the skins.

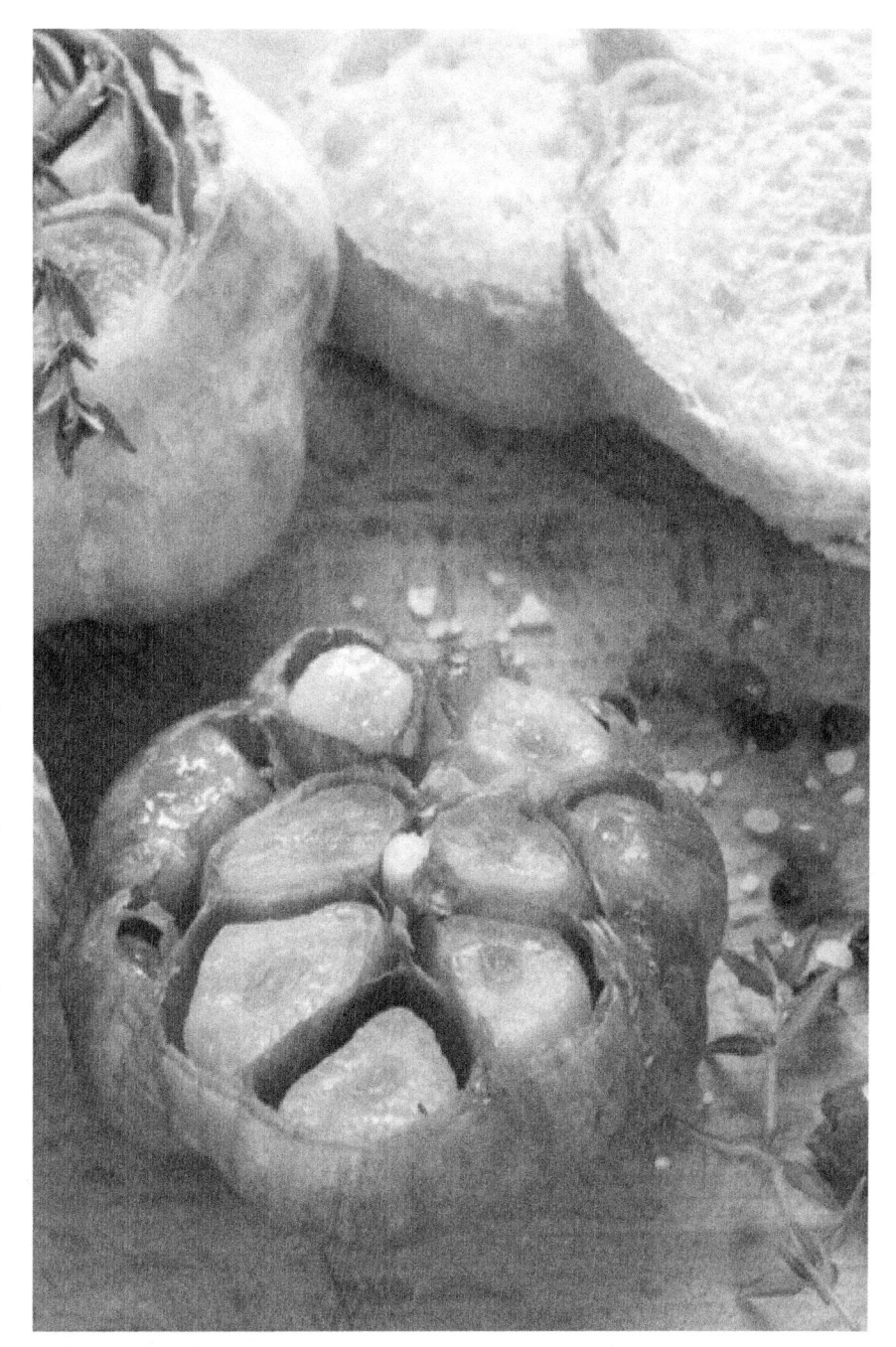

Recipe Notes:
1. You can use just one bulb of garlic if you'd prefer, I do more at once and then store extras in the freezer.
2. Once cooked open the foil and check the garlic, it should be very soft and lightly golden brown. Large bulbs may need a little bit of extra cooking time.
3. Roasted garlic can be used right from frozen, it softens quickly.
4. Keep leftover roasted garlic cloves in the bulb & cover them in the refrigerator for up to 1 week.
5. Freeze roasted garlic by squeezing out the cloves from the skins and then freezing them in a zip-top bag for up to 4 months.

NUTRITION FACTS

Calories: 84, Carbohydrates: 1g, Protein: 1g, Fat: 9g, Saturated Fat: 1g, Polyunsaturated Fat: 1g, Monounsaturated Fat: 7g, Sodium: 1mg, Potassium: 4mg, Fiber: 1g, Sugar: 1g, Vitamin A: 1IU, Vitamin C: 1mg, Calcium: 2mg, Iron: 1mg

Air Fryer Chicken Breasts

PREP TIME: 5 minutes Serves: 4
COOK TIME: 16 minutes
TOTAL TIME: 21 minutes

3

Air Fryer Chicken Breasts are perfectly seasoned, tender & juicy!

- 4 boneless chicken breasts 6-7 oz each
- 1 tablespoon olive oil

Seasoning Mix (or use your favorite seasoning blend)

- ½ teaspoon paprika
- ½ teaspoon garlic powder
- ¼ teaspoon each salt and pepper
- ¼ teaspoon oregano

1. Preheat air fryer to 370°F. Combine the seasoning mix.
2. Rub chicken breasts with olive oil. Season with the mix or your favorite seasoning blend.
3. Place chicken breasts in the air fryer (ensuring they don't overlap) and cook for 10 minutes.
4. Flip chicken over and cook an additional 6-9 minutes or until chicken reaches 165°F. Do not overcook.
5. Rest 5 minutes before slicing.

Recipe Notes:

1. For best results, use an instant-read thermometer to ensure chicken reaches 165°F. Do not overcook.
2. Cook time can vary slightly based on the size/shape of chicken, this recipe is written for 6-7 oz chicken breasts. Chicken breasts can range in size from 5oz to 10oz and appliances can vary. Adjust cook time as needed.
3. Other seasoning options include garlic powder with Italian seasoning, Greek seasoning blend, cajun seasoning or lemon pepper.

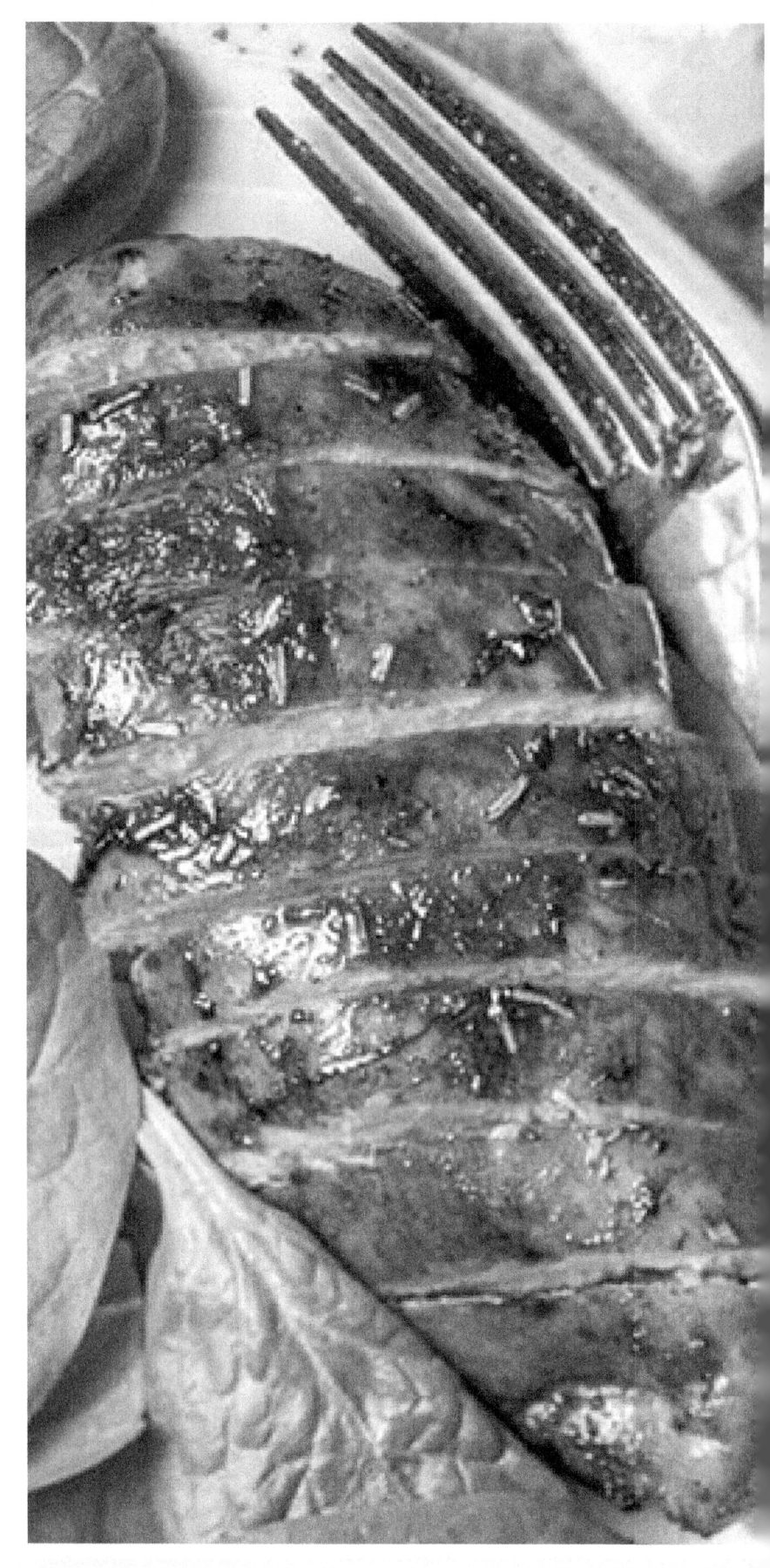

NUTRITION FACTS

Calories: 174, Carbohydrates: 1g, Protein: 24g, Fat: 8g, Saturated Fat: 1g, Cholesterol: 72mg, Sodium: 132mg, Potassium: 418mg, Fiber: 1g, Sugar: 1g, Vitamin A: 69IU, Vitamin C: 1mg, Calcium: 19mg, Iron: 1mg

Air Fryer Pork Tenderloin

PREP TIME: 5 minutes
COOK TIME: 19 minutes
TOTAL TIME: 24 minutes
Serves: 4

Air Fryer Pork tenderloin cooks up juicy and tender every time.

- 1 pork tenderloin about 1 ¼ to 1 ½ pounds
- ½ teaspoon kosher salt
- ¼ teaspoon pepper

Seasoning Mix
- 1 teaspoon dijon mustard
- 1 tablespoon balsamic vinegar
- 1 teaspoon olive oil
- ½ teaspoon Italian seasoning

1. Preheat the air fryer to 400°F.
2. Remove the silver skin from the pork tenderloin by slipping a knife under it. Gently pull the silver area off while cutting with the knife.
3. Combine the seasoning mix in a small bowl and brush over the tenderloin on all sides. Season with salt and pepper.
4. Place the pork tenderloin in the air fryer basket (cut it in half to fit if needed) and cook for 16-17 minutes or until pork reaches 145°F. (I remove the pork from the air fryer a few degrees before as it will continue to rise while resting).
5. Let pork rest at least 5 minutes before serving.

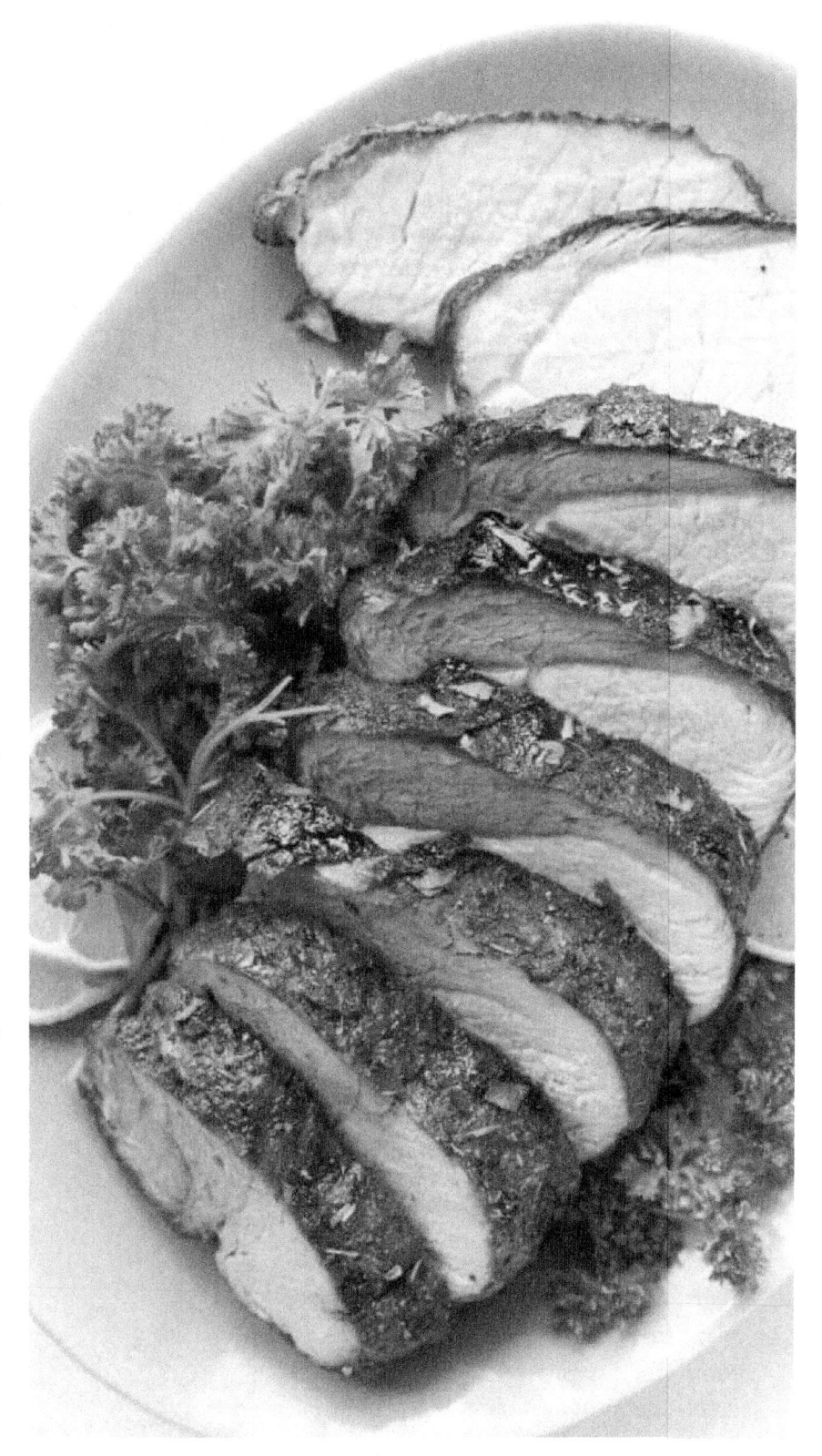

NUTRITION FACTS

Calories: 167, Carbohydrates: 1g, Protein: 30g, Fat: 31g, Saturated Fat: 1g, Polyunsaturated Fat: 1g, Monounsaturated Fat: 1g, Sodium: 306mg, Potassium: 11mg, Fiber: 1g, Sugar: 1g, Vitamin A: 6IU, Vitamin C: 1mg, Calcium: 7mg, Iron: 1mg

Bacon Wrapped Green Bean Bundles

PREP TIME: 10 minutes
COOK TIME: 30 minutes
TOTAL TIME: 40 minutes
Serves: 12

2

Tender crisp green beans wrapped in bacon and brushed with a simple brown sugar glaze are easy enough for a weeknight meal and elegant enough for the holiday table!

- 6 slices bacon
- 1 ½ pounds green beans 6-8 beans per bundle
- ½ teaspoon baking soda
- ¼ teaspoon garlic powder
- salt & pepper to taste
- 1 tablespoon brown sugar

1. Preheat oven to 375°F.
2. Cook bacon on the stovetop until slightly cooked (not crispy), about 3-4 minutes. Reserve any drippings.
3. Trim and wash green beans. Bring a large pot of water to a boil, add baking soda. Add green beans and cook 3 minutes until tender-crisp. Remove from boiling water and place in a bowl of ice water to stop cooking.
4. Dab beans dry and toss with reserved bacon drippings (about 2 teaspoons) or olive oil if you don't have drippings, garlic powder, and salt & pepper to taste.
5. Cut each slice of bacon in half and wrap around about 6-8 green beans, secure with a toothpick, and place on a parchment-lined pan.
6. Combine brown sugar with 1 tablespoon of water and lightly brush over each bundle.
7. Roast 20-22 minutes or until bacon is crisp and beans are lightly roasted.

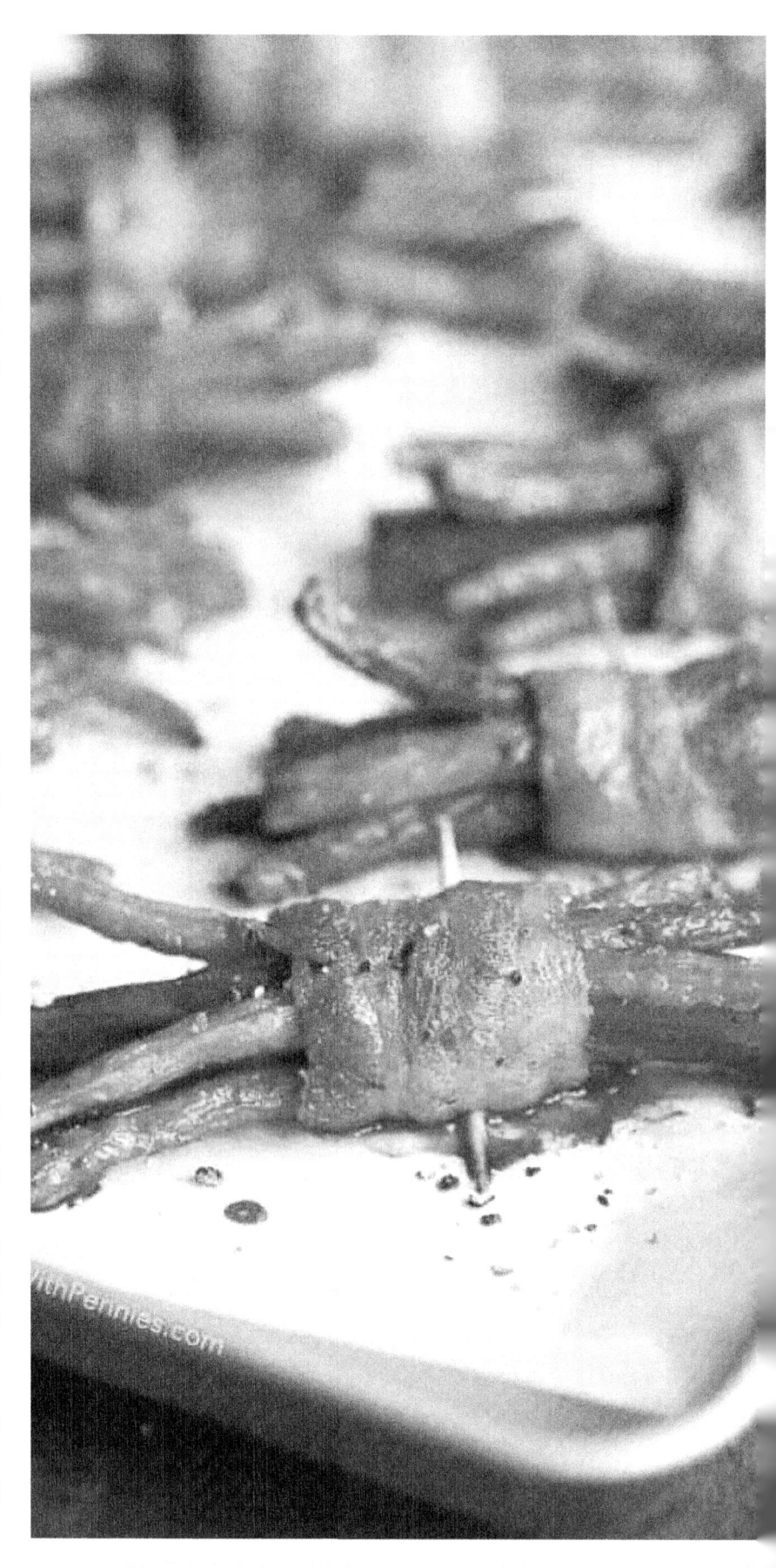

NUTRITION FACTS

Serving: 1bundle, Calories: 67, Carbohydrates: 5g, Protein: 2g, Fat: 4g, Saturated Fat: 1g, Cholesterol: 7mg, Sodium: 122mg, Potassium: 141mg, Fiber: 1g, Sugar: 2g, Vitamin A: 390IU, Vitamin C: 6.9mg, Calcium: 21mg, Iron: 0.6mg

Air Fryer Bacon Wrapped Brussels Sprouts

PREP TIME: 12 minutes
COOK TIME: 15 minutes
TOTAL TIME: 27 minutes
Serves: 4

`24`

Brussels Sprouts are wrapped in bacon, sprinkled with brown sugar, then air fried until crispy on the outside & tender on the inside!

- 1 pound bacon
- 1 ½ pounds brussels sprouts
- ½ cup brown sugar

1. Preheat the air fryer to 375°F.
2. Wash & trim Brussels sprouts. If they are large, cut them in half.
3. Cut each slice of bacon into thirds and wrap around a sprout.
4. Line the basket with parchment paper (do not preheat with parchment paper). Place seam side down in the basket and sprinkle brown sugar on top. Repeat with remaining brussels & bacon.
5. Bake 15 minutes or until bacon is crisp and brussels sprouts are tender.

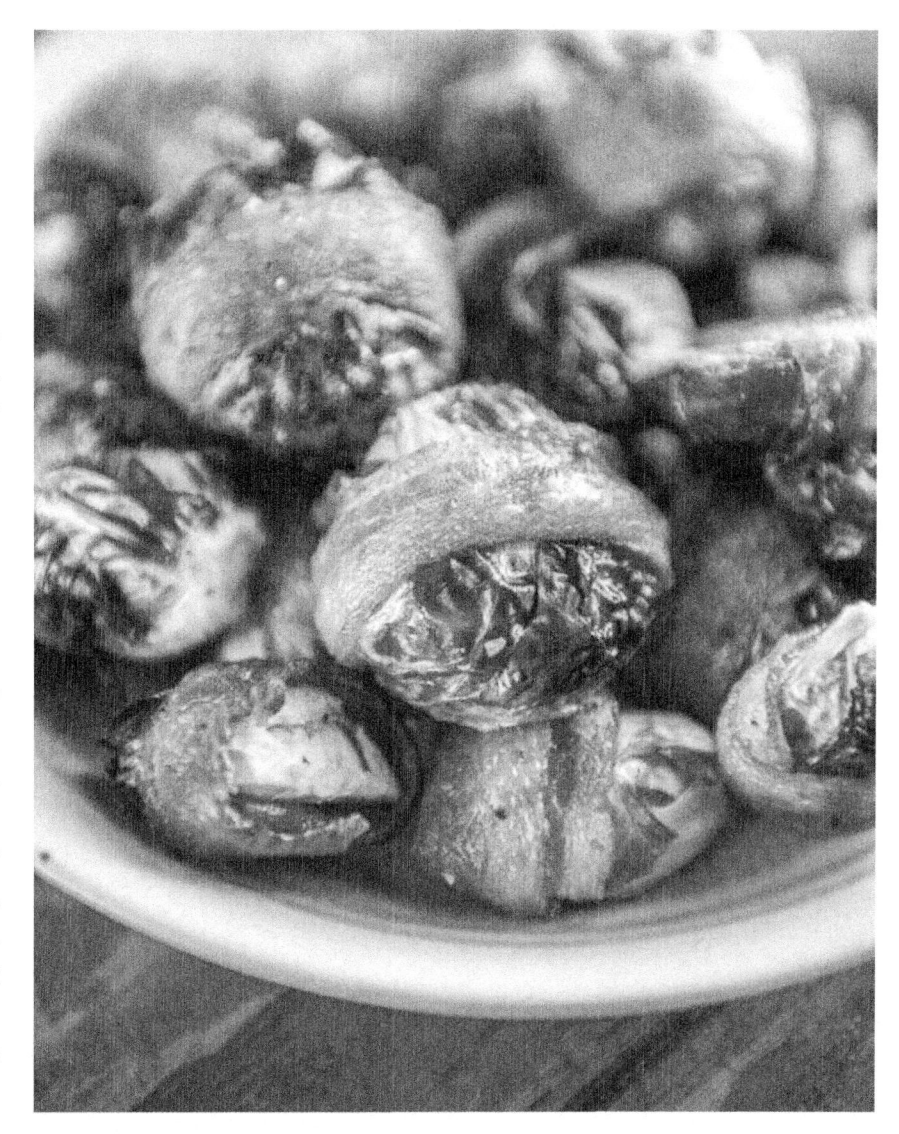

Recipe Notes

1. No Air Fryer? No Problem! These can be baked in the oven at 425°F for about 22-27 minutes or until bacon is crisp and Brussels sprouts are tender.
2. Do not preheat the air fryer with parchment paper or it will blow around and burn.
3. Thick-cut bacon should need to be partially cooked before wrapping. Air fry thick cut bacon for 3-4 minutes or just until softened and cool slightly before wrapping. Regular cut bacon doesn't need to be partially cooked.
4. If the Brussels are large, cut them in half.
5. If using frozen Brussels, they do not need to be thawed but the cooking time will need to be increased.
6. Cook them seam side down so the bacon does not unravel.
7. Brussels can be prepared 48 hours in advance and cooked before serving.
8. Don't crowd the basket. The more airflow, the crispier the Brussels will be. Cook in batches if needed.
9. Store leftovers in an airtight container in the refrigerator for 3-5 days. They can also be frozen and will last in the freezer for 3 months.
10. Reheat in the air fryer at 350°F for 10 minutes or until heated through.

NUTRITION FACTS

Calories: 651, Carbohydrates: 44g, Protein: 20g, Fat: 46g, Saturated Fat: 15g, Polyunsaturated Fat: 8g, Monounsaturated Fat: 20g, Trans Fat: 1g, Cholesterol: 75mg, Sodium: 801mg, Potassium: 923mg, Fiber: 6g, Sugar: 30g, Vitamin A: 1324IU, Vitamin C: 145mg, Calcium: 100mg, Iron: 3mg

Chapter 6:
Beverage

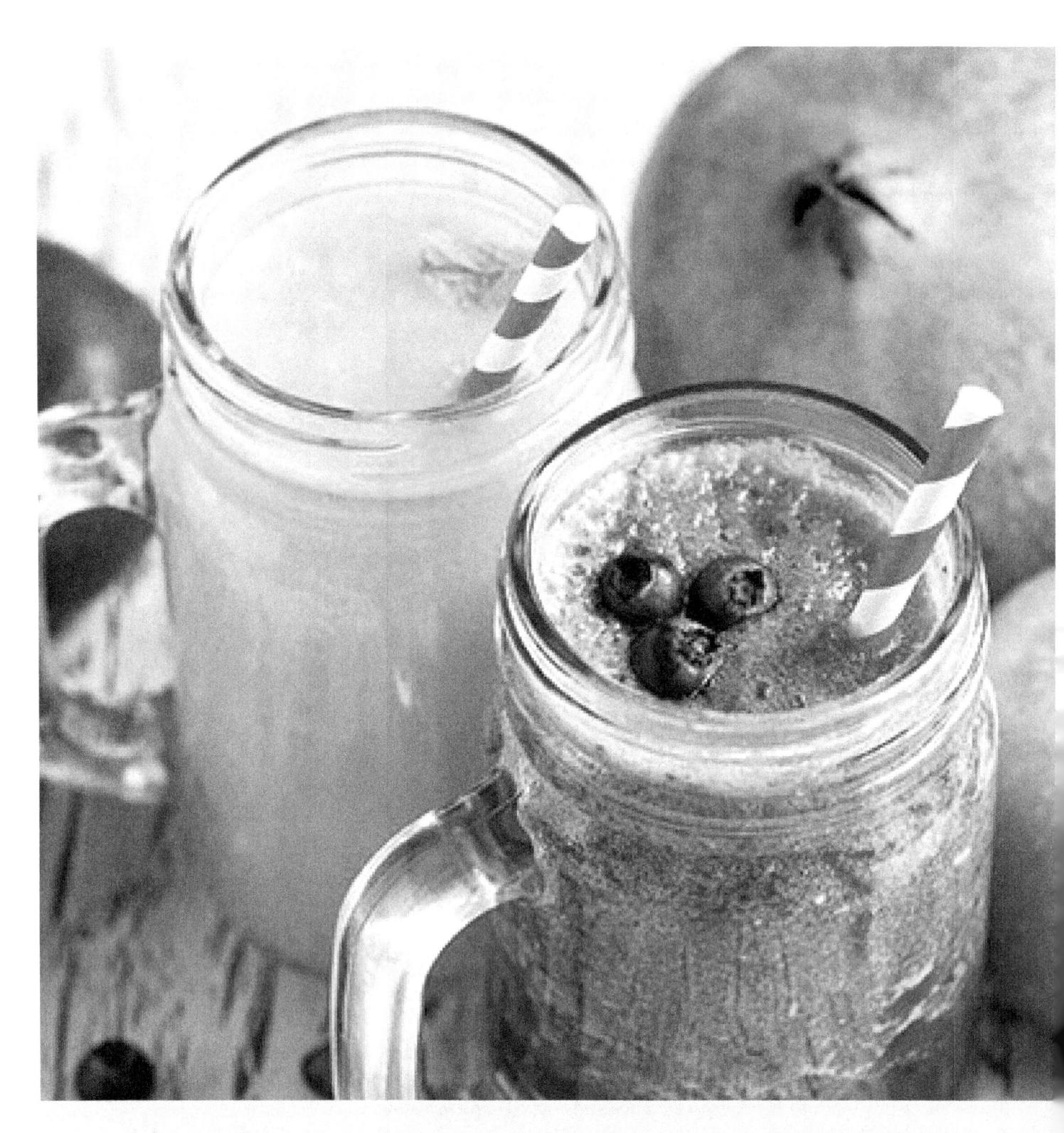

Copycat Baileys Recipe (Homemade Irish Cream)

PREP TIME: 5 minutes   Serves: 12
CHILL TIME: 1 day
TOTAL TIME: 1 day 5 minutes

8

Baileys Irish Cream is creamy & flavorful with a bit of a kick. The best part is, this copycat recipe is ready in under 5 minutes!

- 1 can sweetened condensed milk 14 ounces
- 2 cups light cream or half and half
- 1 cup whiskey
- 1 teaspoon instant coffee granules
- 1 teaspoon vanilla extract

1. Combine all ingredients in jar with a tight-fitting lid.
2. Shake to mix well. Chill at least 24 hours before serving.
3. Store in the refrigerator up to 2 weeks.

Recipe Notes:
1. This Irish cream can be made without alcohol. Skip the whiskey and add a teaspoon or so of rum or whiskey extract. While the flavor is slightly different, it's delicious!
2. This will keep in the fridge as long as the expiry date on your cream.
3. Serve over ice, in cocktails, or in coffee.

Nutrition Facts
Per Serving: Calories: 215, Carbohydrates: 19g, Protein: 3g, Fat: 9g, Saturated Fat: 6g, Cholesterol: 33mg, Sodium: 49mg, Potassium: 145mg, Sugar: 18g, Vitamin A: 291IU, Vitamin C: 1mg, Calcium: 108mg, Iron: 1mg

Easy Mulled Wine Recipe

PREP TIME 5 minutes   Serves: 5
COOK TIME 20 minutes
TOTAL TIME 25 minutes

4

Sweet, savory, and served warm from the stovetop, this Mulled Wine is a perfect way to celebrate the holidays!

- 750 ml red wine any wine you'd like
- 6 whole cloves
- 3 cinnamon sticks
- 3 allspice berries optional
- 1 orange sliced
- ¼ cup honey more or less to taste
- cranberries for garnish
- candied orange slices for garnish
- rosemary sprig for garnish

1. Combine wine and spices in a medium saucepan.
2. Add orange slices and honey and heat over low heat for 20 minutes. Do not simmer.
3. To serve, place the mulled wine in mugs and garnish as desired. We add cranberries, orange slices, and rosemary or a cinnamon stick.

Nutrition Facts
Serving: 5oz, Calories: 185, Carbohydrates: 20g, Protein: 1g, Fat: 1g, Saturated Fat: 1g, Polyunsaturated Fat: 1g, Monounsaturated Fat: 1g, Sodium: 8mg, Potassium: 211mg, Fiber: 1g, Sugar: 15g, Vitamin A: 10IU, Vitamin C: 1mg, Calcium: 36mg, Iron: 1mg

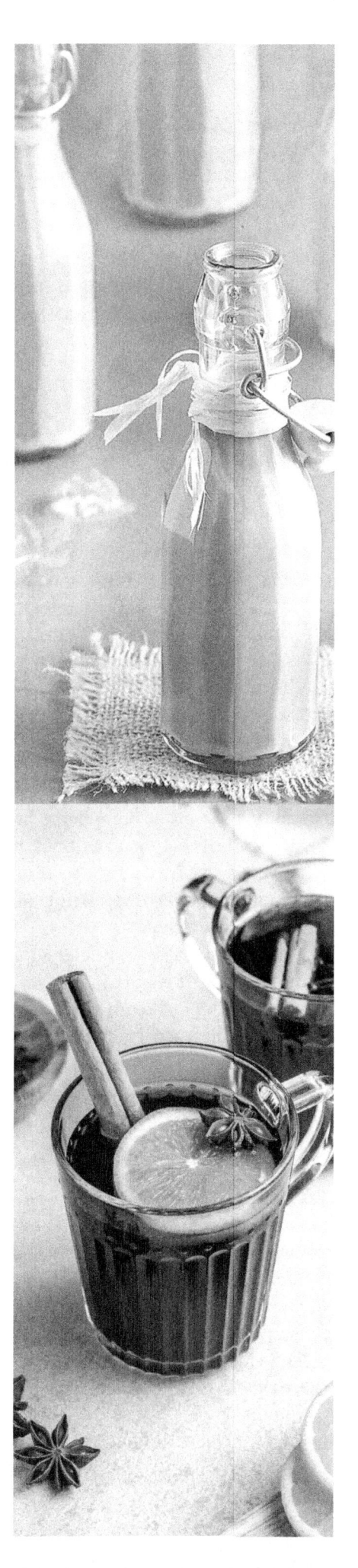

Green Kiwi Smoothie

PREP TIME: 5 minutes Serves: 2
COOK TIME: 5 minutes
TOTAL TIME: 10 minutes

6

A handful of fresh fruit & veggies, some yogurt, & a bit of honey makes this smoothie creamy, flavorful, and totally irresistible!

- ¼ cup kale optional
- ¼ cup orange juice
- ⅓ cup yogurt
- 4 kiwis
- 1 cup pineapple
- 1 cup ice
- 1-2 teaspoons honey

1. Place kale, orange juice, and yogurt in a blender and blend until smooth.
2. Add remaining ingredients and blend until smooth.
3. Serve immediately.

Recipe Notes :
1. Blending the kale with juice before adding the other ingredients helps it to be fully blended and smooth.
2. Use fresh fruit for a thinner smoothie and frozen fruit for a thicker smoothie.
3. You can use sweetened or unsweetened yogurt in this recipe. If using plain yogurt, you might need to increase the honey to taste.
4. Leftovers can be frozen in ice cube trays and added to future smoothies.

Nutrition Facts

Per Serving: Calories: 197,
Carbohydrates: 44g, Protein: 5g, Fat: 3g,
Saturated Fat: 1g, Polyunsaturated Fat: 1g, Monounsaturated Fat: 1g,
Cholesterol: 5mg, Sodium: 35mg,
Potassium: 824mg, Fiber: 7g, Sugar: 29g,
Vitamin A: 1145IU, Vitamin C: 234mg,
Calcium: 142mg, Iron: 1mg

Bahama Mama

PREP TIME: 5 minutes Serves: 1
TOTAL TIME: 5 minutes

3

This tropical cocktail is made with dark rum, Kahlua, coconut rum, pineapple juice, orange juice, and grenadine for a fun, fruity, and dangerously boozy drink!

- 1 ounce coconut rum
- 1 ounce pineapple juice
- 1 ounce orange juice
- ½ ounce dark rum
- ¼ ounce Kahlua
- ½ ounce grenadine
- splash of club soda optional
- orange slice for garnish
- Maraschino cherry for garnish

1. Add coconut rum, pineapple juice, orange juice, dark rum, and Kahlua to a cocktail shaker with ice and shake vigorously for 15 seconds until chilled.
2. Strain into a glass filled with ice and slowly pour in the grenadine and top with club soda.
3. Garnish with an orange slice and maraschino cherry and drink as is or stir.

Recipe Notes
1. If you would prefer a non-layered look, you can add the grenadine directly to the shaker with the other ingredients.
2. Do not add club soda to the shaker since it's carbonated.
3. ½ ounce of lemon juice may be added to the drink for a more vibrant cocktail.

Nutrition Facts

Calories: 188, Carbohydrates: 19g, Protein: 1g, Fat: 1g, Saturated Fat: 1g, Sodium: 6mg,
Potassium: 98mg, Fiber: 1g, Sugar: 15g,
Vitamin A: 58IU, Vitamin C: 17mg,
Calcium: 8mg, Iron: 1mg

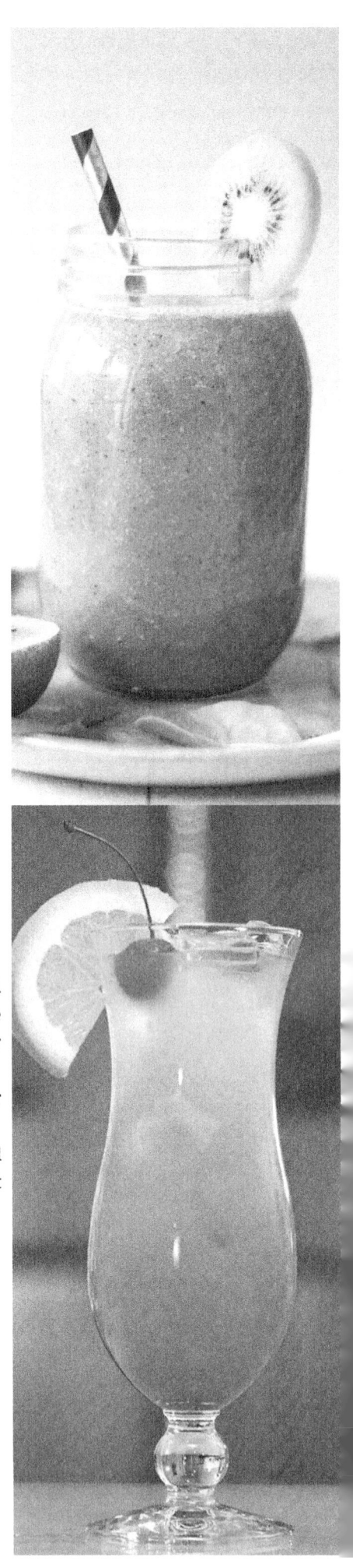

Easy Red Sangria

PREP TIME: 15 minutes   Serves: 4
COOK TIME: 5 minutes
CHILL TIME: 1 hour
TOTAL TIME: 1 hour 20 minutes

6

Colorful, bright, & refreshing, this Red Sangria is a fruity drink you didn't know you needed!

- 2 limes divided (one juiced, one sliced)
- 2 lemons divided (one juiced, one sliced)
- 1 bottle red wine 750ml
- ½ cup orange juice
- ½ cup apricot brandy
- ¼ cup simple syrup or to taste
- 2 ounces triple sec
- 1 orange sliced
- 1 apple sliced
- 2 cups club soda or lemon-lime soda, optional

1. Juice one lemon and one lime. Slice remaining fruit.
2. In a large pitcher, combine red wine, lime juice, lemon juice, orange juice, brandy, simple syrup, triple sec, and sliced fruit.
3. Refrigerate at least 1 hour.
4. To serve, fill a glass with ice and fill ⅔ of the way with sangria. Top with soda as desired.

Nutrition Facts
Per Serving: Calories: 401, Carbohydrates: 45g, Protein: 1g, Fat: 1g, Saturated Fat: 1g, Sodium: 48mg, Potassium: 521mg, Fiber: 4g, Sugar: 33g, Vitamin A: 183IU, Vitamin C: 68mg, Calcium: 59mg, Iron: 2mg

Tequila Sunrise

PREP TIME: 5 minutes   Serves: 2
TOTAL TIME: 5 minutes

3

Sweet, tart, and super refreshing, this Tequila Sunrise is the perfect cocktail to enjoy with friends!

- 4 ounces tequila
- 8 ounces orange juice
- 1 ounce grenadine
- oranges and cherries for garnish

1. Fill two medium glasses with ice.
2. Divide tequila and orange juice over the two glasses.
3. Gently top with grenadine.
4. Garnish with oranges and cherries.

Recipe Notes
1. Chill glasses in freezer for best results.

Nutrition Facts
Calories: 220, Carbohydrates: 21g, Protein: 1g, Fat: 1g, Saturated Fat: 1g, Sodium: 6mg, Potassium: 232mg, Fiber: 1g, Sugar: 16g, Vitamin A: 227IU, Vitamin C: 57mg, Calcium: 13mg, Iron: 1mg

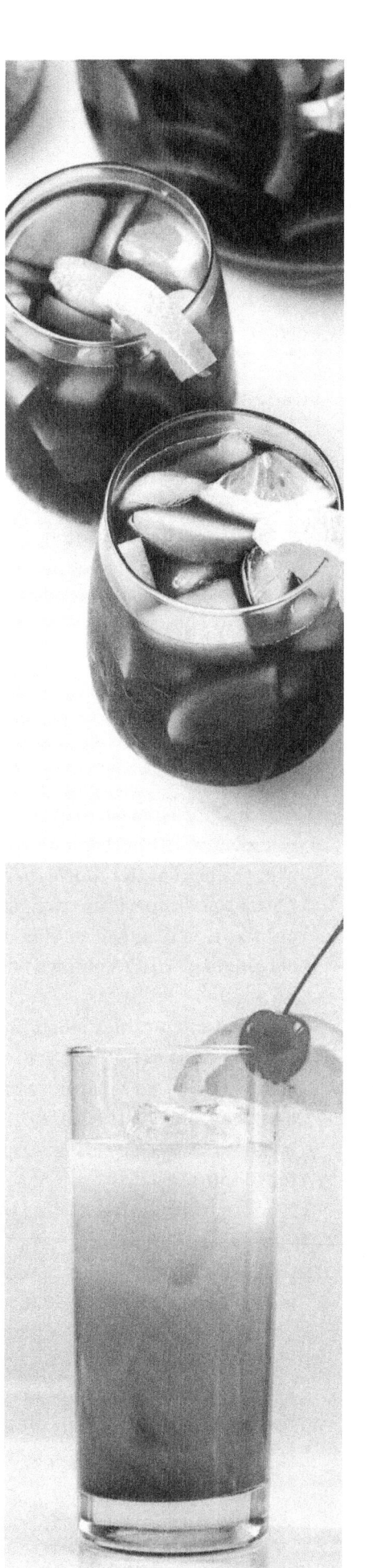

Hot Chocolate Bombs

PREP TIME: 1 hour
COOL TIME: 15 minutes
TOTAL TIME: 1 hour 15 minutes
Serves: 6

5

Made with just 3 ingredients, these chocolate bombs will result in a creamy and decadent mug of hot chocolate when you add steaming hot milk to them!

- 12 ounces couverture chocolate morsels or finely chopped high-quality chocolate such as Ghirardelli baking chocolate, divided - see notes
- 6 hot chocolate mix packets between .85 oz. and 1.25 oz. in size
- mini marshmallows
- sprinkles optional
- 8 ounces whole milk or milk of choice for serving

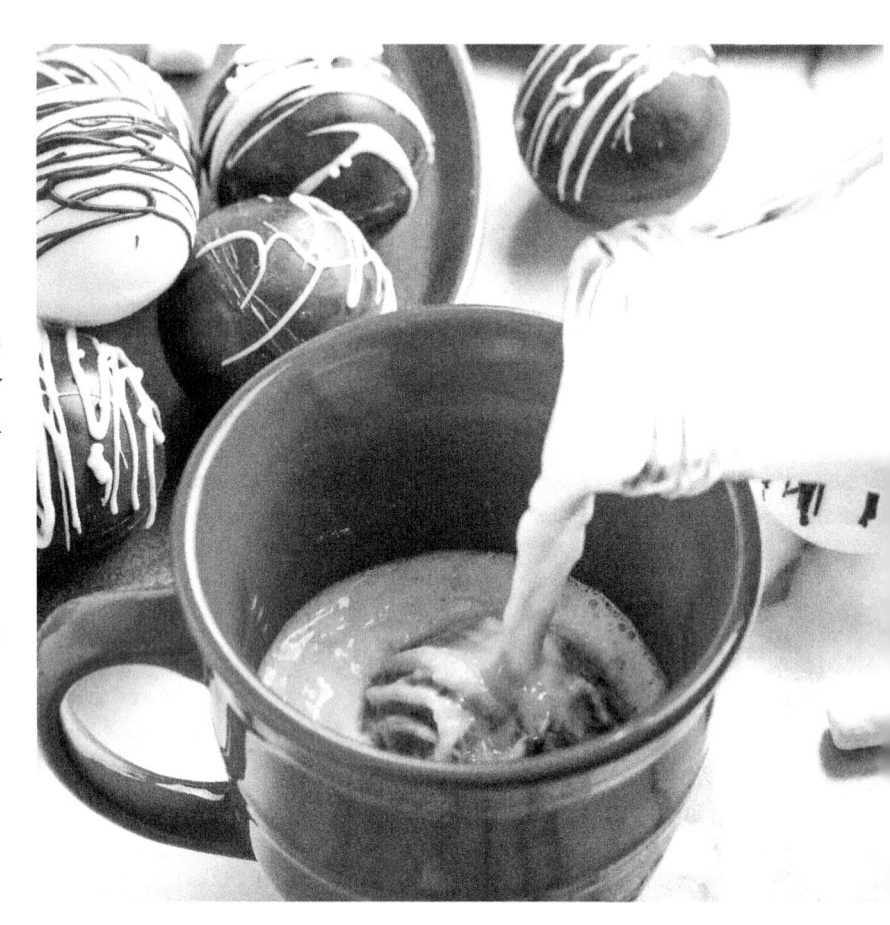

Melt Chocolate
1. Add 5 ounces of chocolate to a medium bowl and microwave for 30 seconds, remove and stir. Continue to microwave at 15-second intervals stirring until almost melted (there should be some bits left). Continue to stir so that the heat of the chocolate melts the unmelted pieces.
2. Check the temperature to make sure that the chocolate reads 88-90°F. If the temperature is over 90 degrees, stir in an additional ounce of chocolate until melted to bring it to between 88-90 degrees. This process ensures the chocolate is shiny & glossy and sets firm.

Create Shells
1. Spoon about 1 tablespoon of melted chocolate into each mold and use the back of the spoon to spread it around make sure to get all the way to the top of the rim and not leave any exposed areas. Place the mold on the small baking sheet and refrigerate for 5 minutes.
2. Remove from the refrigerator and spoon another heaping spoonful into one of the molds and spread it as a second layer. Be sure to do this one at a time or the chocolate will cool too quickly before you get to spread it on each. Freeze for 10 minutes.
3. Remove from the freezer and put food-safe gloves. Remove the chocolate shells from the molds.

Fill Shells & Seal
1. Once all of your shells are made, microwave a plate for minutes. Half of the shells, open side down, on the warm plate and gently spin them to smooth the edge.
2. Place the shells in a cupcake liner (or pan) open side up and fill the cavities with a packet of hot cocoa mix and marshmallows.
3. Reheat the plate for 2 minutes in the microwave. One at a time, place a shell open side down to melt the edge and then place it on top of one of the filled shells to seal. Run your finger along the edge to smooth it.
4. Let the hot chocolate bombs chill for a few minutes to set. Top with a drizzle of chocolate and sprinkles if desired.

NUTRITION FACTS

Calories: 107, Carbohydrates: 23g, Protein: 1g, Fat: 2g, Saturated Fat: 2g, Trans Fat: 1g, Sodium: 139mg, Potassium: 1mg, Fiber: 1g, Sugar: 18g, Vitamin A: 2IU, Calcium: 15mg, Iron: 1mg

Copycat Shamrock Shake Recipe

PREP TIME: 5 minutes Serves: 2
TOTAL TIME: 5 minutes

25

These light & creamy Shamrock Shakes are the perfect way to celebrate St. Patrick's Day!

- 4 cups vanilla ice cream
- ¼ cup milk
- ½ tsp peppermint extract or more to taste
- green food coloring
- toppings like whipped cream, cherries, & sprinkles for garnish

1. Combine all ingredients in a blender and blend until smooth.
2. Garnish as desired and serve immediately.

Recipe Notes

1. For a healthy-ish version, use vanilla frozen yogurt and swap the liquid for fat-free milk, and omit the whipped cream.
2. Spike this favorite with a splash of creme de menthe, Baileys, or vodka for a boozy treat!

Nutrition Facts
Per Serving: Calories: 562, Carbohydrates: 64g, Protein: 10g, Fat: 29g, Saturated Fat: 18g, Cholesterol: 118mg, Sodium: 224mg, Potassium: 571mg, Fiber: 2g, Sugar: 58g, Vitamin A: 1169IU, Vitamin C: 2mg, Calcium: 375mg, Iron: 1mg

Snickerdoodle Cocktail (with RumChata)

PREP TIME: 5 minutes Serves: 1
TOTAL TIME: 5 minutes

11

This creamy cocktail tastes like snickerdoodle cookies or a cinnamon vanilla milkshake. It's made with RumChata, Amaretto, milk, and Buttershots that give it that irresistible cookie essence!

- Ice
- 1 ½ ounces RumChata
- 1 ounce whole milk
- ½ ounce Amaretto
- ½ ounce Buttershots
- 2 teaspoons simple syrup for rim
- 2 tablespoons cinnamon sugar for rim
- cinnamon stick for garnish

1. Add ice to a cocktail shaker and pour in the RumChata, milk, Amaretto, and Buttershots. Cover and shake vigorously for 15 seconds.
2. Dip the rim of a cocktail glass in the simple syrup and then in the cinnamon sugar, moving it around to coat.
3. Strain the drink into the prepared cocktail glass, garnish with a cinnamon stick, and serve immediately.

Recipe Notes

1. This is also really delicious hot with an additional 4 ounces of milk and topped with whipped cream. Heat the milk on the stove and then add in the liquor

Nutrition Facts
Calories: 381, Carbohydrates: 65g, Protein: 1g, Fat: 1g, Saturated Fat: 1g, Cholesterol: 3mg, Sodium: 26mg, Potassium: 37mg, Sugar: 65g, Calcium: 32mg, Iron: 1mg

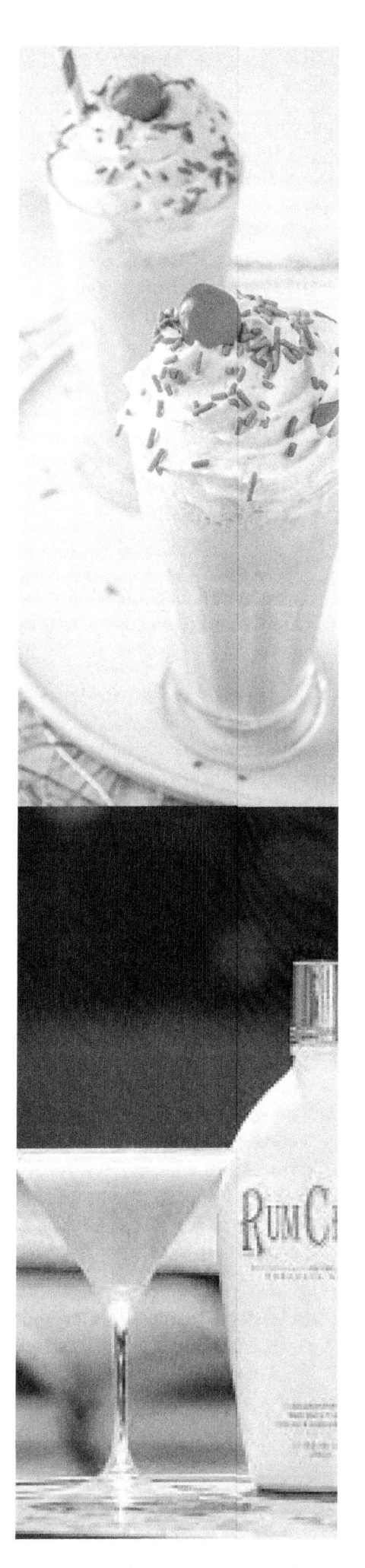

Champagne Punch

PREP TIME: 10 minutes Serves: 2
COOK TIME: 5 minutes
TOTAL TIME: 15 minutes

5

This Cranberry Champagne Punch is loaded with fresh fruit and mint leaves. It's the perfect cocktail for a holiday get-together!

- 3 cups pomegranate juice
- 2 cups ginger ale or club soda (or to taste)
- 1 cup orange juice
- ⅓ cup triple sec or Cointreau
- 1 ½ tablespoons lime juice
- 750 milliliters champagne or sparkling wine
- ice and fruit for garnish limes, fresh cranberries, pomegranate arils and mint

1. Combine pomegranate juice, ginger ale, orange juice, triple sec, and lime juice in a drink pitcher. Cover and refrigerate up to 24 hours.
2. Fill cocktail glasses ⅔ full with the juice mixture (about 6 ounces). Add ice and top with champagne or sparkling wine (about 3 ounces).
3. Garnish with cranberries, mint, and pomegranate arils.

Recipe Notes
1. For a sweeter cocktail, add some simple syrup or additional gingerale.
2. To make festive ice cubes, place fruit (cranberries/lime/mint) in the bottom of an ice cube tray. Fill the cubes ⅓ with water and freeze. Once frozen, fill the tray the rest of the way with water and freeze. This keeps the fruit from floating to the top of the ice.

Nutrition Facts
Calories: 161, Carbohydrates: 25g, Protein: 1g, Fat: 1g, Saturated Fat: 1g, Sodium: 20mg, Potassium: 344mg, Fiber: 1g, Sugar: 24g, Vitamin A: 62IU, Vitamin C: 16mg, Calcium: 24mg, Iron: 1mg

Kale Smoothie

PREP TIME: 5 minutes Serves: 2
COOK TIME: 5 minutes
TOTAL TIME: 10 minutes

14

This Kale Smoothie is healthy, full of fresh fruits & veggies, and makes the perfect snack!

- 3 cups kale chopped
- 1 cup plain yogurt or vanilla yogurt
- 1 ¼ cup orange juice or as needed
- 2 bananas frozen
- 1 cup frozen fruit of your choice I prefer pineapple, strawberry, or peach
- 2 teaspoons honey or preferred sweetener

1. Blend kale, yogurt and orange juice until smooth.
2. Add remaining ingredients and blend until smooth.
3. Divide over two glasses and serve immediately.

Nutrition Facts
Calories: 388, Carbohydrates: 81g, Protein: 11g, Fat: 6g, Saturated Fat: 3g, Cholesterol: 16mg, Sodium: 103mg, Potassium: 1521mg, Fiber: 5g, Sugar: 52g, Vitamin A: 10905IU, Vitamin C: 212mg, Calcium: 328mg, Iron: 2mg

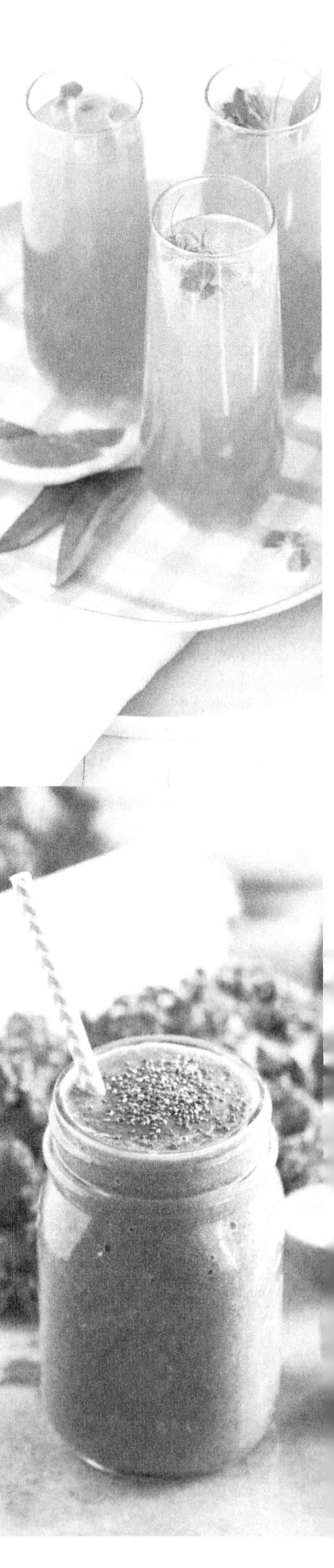

Blueberry Smoothie

COOK TIME: 5 minutes Serves: 2
TOTAL TIME: 5 minutes

8

Blueberry Smoothies are healthy, hearty, and ready in 5 minutes!

- 2 cups fresh or frozen blueberries
- 1 cup milk
- ½ cup vanilla yogurt
- 1 banana frozen, cut into chunks

1. Add all ingredients to a blender.
2. Blend until smooth.
3. Serve immediately.

Nutrition Facts

Calories: 238, Carbohydrates: 49g, Protein: 9g, Fat: 3g, Saturated Fat: 1g, Cholesterol: 9mg, Sodium: 94mg, Potassium: 636mg, Fiber: 5g, Sugar: 37g, Vitamin A: 375IU, Vitamin C: 20mg, Calcium: 261mg, Iron: 1mg

Fresh Homemade Limeade

PREP TIME: 5 minutes Serves: 16
COOK TIME: 5 minutes
TOTAL TIME: 10 minutes

3

This homemade limeade recipe is sweet and tangy and makes enough to share!

- 2 cups water
- 1 cup sugar
- 1 cup fresh lime juice
- 1 teaspoon lime zest about 1 lime
- water for serving

1. Combine 2 cups water, sugar and lime juice in a saucepan.
2. Stir over medium heat until sugar is completely dissolved. Cool completely.
3. Stir in lime zest. Store in the fridge up to 1 week.

To Make Limeade
1. Combine equal parts lime juice mixture and water over ice.

Nutrition Facts

Serving: 1cup, Calories: 52, Carbohydrates: 14g, Protein: 1g, Fat: 1g, Saturated Fat: 1g, Sodium: 2mg, Potassium: 18mg, Fiber: 1g, Sugar: 13g, Vitamin A: 8IU, Vitamin C: 5mg, Calcium: 3mg, Iron: 1mg

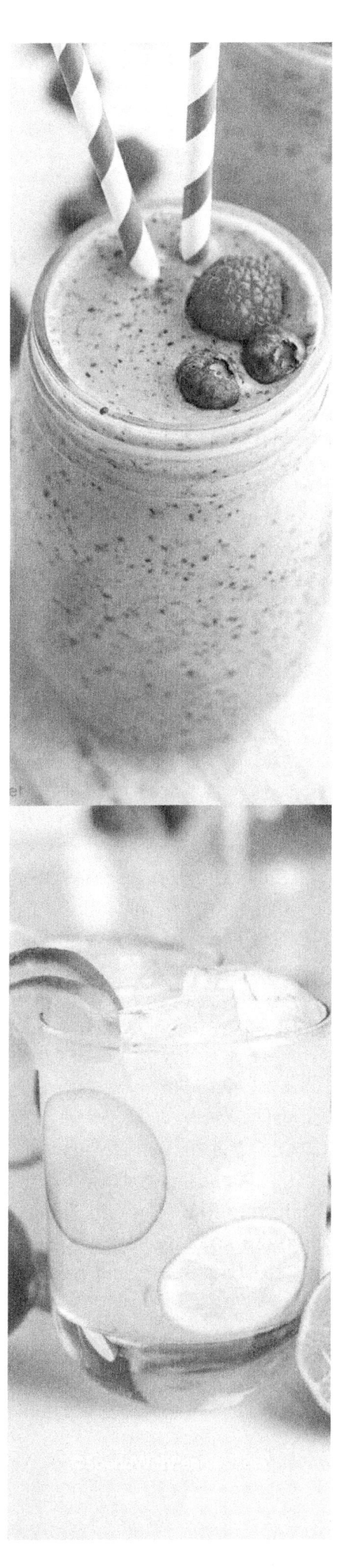

Whipped Coffee (Dalgona)

PREP TIME: 10 minutes   Serves: 1
COOK TIME: 5 minutes
TOTAL TIME: 15 minutes

5

Whether it's served hot or cold, this creamy dreamy whipped coffee is an easy and decadent treat!

- 1 tablespoon instant coffee
- 1 tablespoon sugar
- 1 tablespoon hot water
- 6 ounces milk for serving

1. Combine instant coffee, sugar and water in a medium bowl.
2. Whisk on high with an electric mixer until thick and creamy, about 5-7 minutes.
3. Heat milk on the stove or over the microwave if desired (this can be served over cold milk too). Top with whipped coffee and serve.

Recipe Notes
1. Hot water works best for this recipe.
2. This recipe can be doubled, tripled or more!
3. Leftovers can be frozen or refrigerated.

Nutrition Facts
Calories: 136, Carbohydrates: 24g, Protein: 6g, Fat: 2g, Saturated Fat: 1g, Cholesterol: 9mg, Sodium: 78mg, Potassium: 432mg, Sugar: 21g, Vitamin A: 333IU, Calcium: 213mg, Iron: 1mg

Aperol Spritz

PREP TIME: 10 minutes   Serves: 1
COOK TIME: 0 minutes
TOTAL TIME: 10 minutes

3

This sweet and delicious beverage is made with just 3 ingredients!

- 5 ounces prosecco
- 2 ounces Aperol
- 2 ounces club soda
- ice
- orange slices for garnish

1. Fill a wine glass with ice.
2. Add remaining ingredients.
3. Garnish with orange wedges.

Nutrition Facts
Calories: 163, Carbohydrates: 16g, Protein: 1g, Sodium: 22mg, Potassium: 125mg, Sugar: 16g, Calcium: 13mg, Iron: 1mg

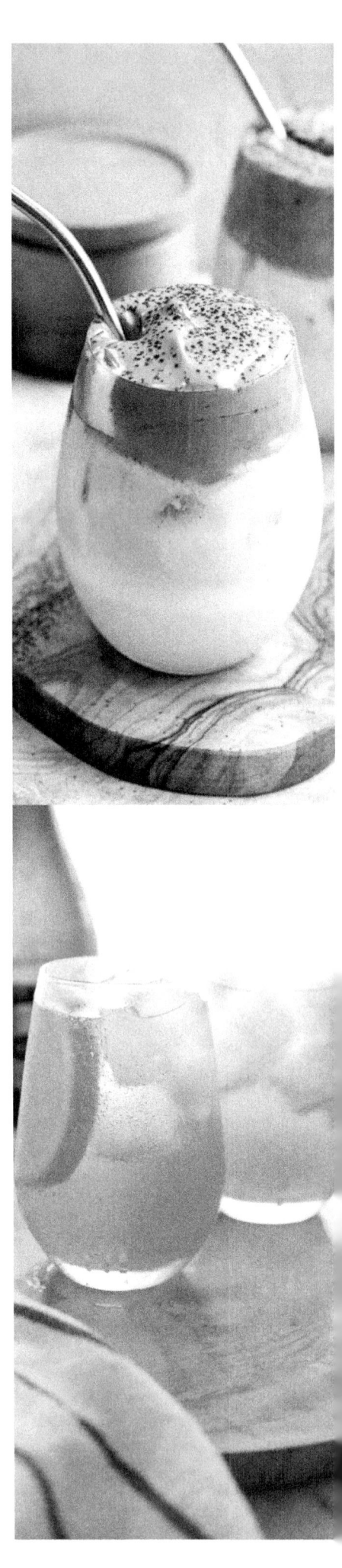

Dark and Stormy Cocktail

PREP TIME: 5 minutes Serves: 1
COOK TIME: 0 minutes
TOTAL TIME: 5 minutes

2

A spicy, heartwarming cocktail that is sure to turn up the heat!

- 4 ounces ginger beer
- 1 ½ ounces Gosling's Black Seal rum (dark rum)
- lime wedges

1. Fill a short glass with ice cubes.
2. Add ginger beer. Slowly add dark rum pouring over an ice cube to get the layered effect.
3. Garnish with a lime wedges and serve.

Recipe Notes
1. Drink should be stirred before serving.

Nutrition Facts
Calories: 137, Carbohydrates: 10g, Sodium: 8mg, Sugar: 10g, Iron: 1mg

Classic Bloody Mary

PREP TIME: 10 minutes Serves: 1
COOK TIME: 0 minutes
TOTAL TIME: 10 minutes

2

Spicy and oh so savory with a refreshing tang!

- celery salt for the rim of the glass optional
- ice cubes
- 1 ½ ounces vodka
- ¾ cup spicy vegetable juice cocktail
- 2 dashes Worcestershire sauce
- pinch of celery salt
- 1 dash tabasco
- 2 teaspoon lemon juice
- 1 stalk celery
- 1 pickled beans optional

1. Moisten the rim of a glass. Pour celery salt onto a shallow plate and rub the glass in the salt. Set aside.
2. Combine all remaining ingredients (except garnisin a cocktail shaker. Top with ice and shake well.
3. Fill the prepared glass with ice and strain tomato mixture into the glass.

Nutrition Facts
Calories: 158, Carbohydrates: 12g, Protein: 2g, Fat: 1g, Saturated Fat: 1g, Sodium: 2314mg, Potassium: 550mg, Fiber: 2g, Sugar: 9g, Vitamin A: 1794IU, Vitamin C: 64mg, Calcium: 58mg, Iron: 2mg

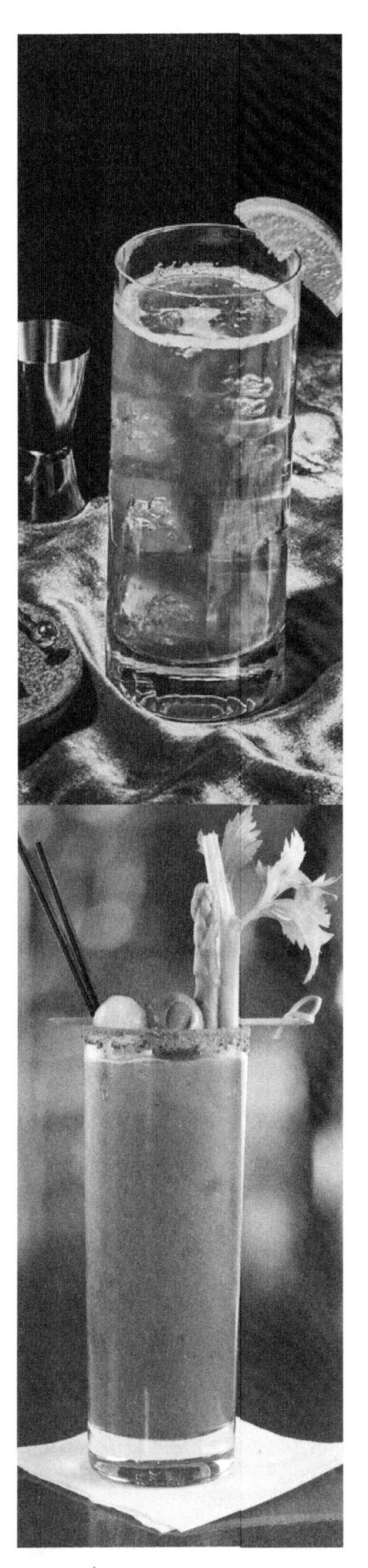

Kir Royale Cocktail

PREP TIME: 5 minutes Serves: 1
COOK TIME: 0 minutes
TOTAL TIME: 5 minutes

2

Fruity and fizzy Kir Royale is a classy cocktail that's delicious and guaranteed to make your guests feel extra special.

- 1 ounce chambord or crème de cassis
- 5 ounces prosecco or sparkling wine
- lemon twist or raspberries

1. Pour chambord into a wine flute.
2. Top with prosecco or sparkling wine.
3. Garnish and serve.

Nutrition Facts
Calories: 157, Carbohydrates: 11g, Protein: 1g, Fat: 1g, Saturated Fat: 1g, Sodium: 12mg, Potassium: 125mg, Sugar: 11g, Calcium: 13mg, Iron: 1mg

Classic Martini Recipe

PREP TIME: 10 minutes Serves: 1
COOK TIME: 0 minutes
TOTAL TIME: 10 minutes

1

An ideal cocktail for New Year's parties or any time of the year!

- 2 ounces vodka
- 1 teaspoon dry vermouth optional
- 2 large pimento stuffed olives
- ice

1. Place martini glasses in the freezer.
2. Fill a cocktail shaker with ice.
3. Add vodka and vermouth, shake very well.
4. Pour a dash of vermouth into the prepared martini glass and swirl it around. Discard the vermouth.
5. Strain vodka into chilled glasses. Add olives and serve immediately.

1. Place martini glasses in the freezer.
2. Fill a cocktail shaker with ice.
3. Add vodka and vermouth, shake very well.
4. Pour a dash of vermouth into the prepared martini glass and swirl it around. Discard the vermouth.
5. Strain vodka into chilled glasses. Add olives and serve immediately.

Nutrition Facts
Calories: 147, Carbohydrates: 1g, Protein: 1g, Fat: 1g, Saturated Fat: 1g, Sodium: 125mg, Fiber: 1g, Sugar: 1g

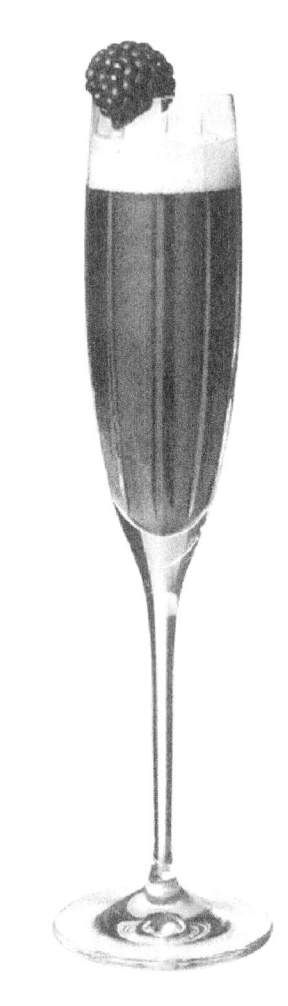

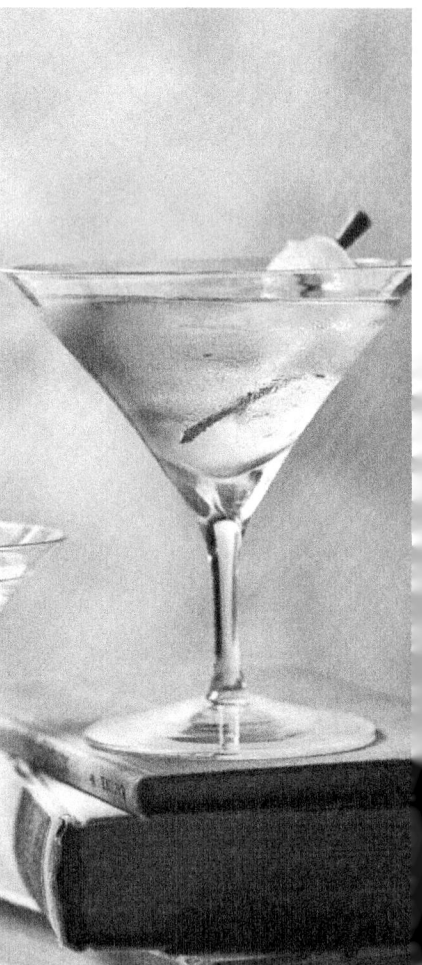

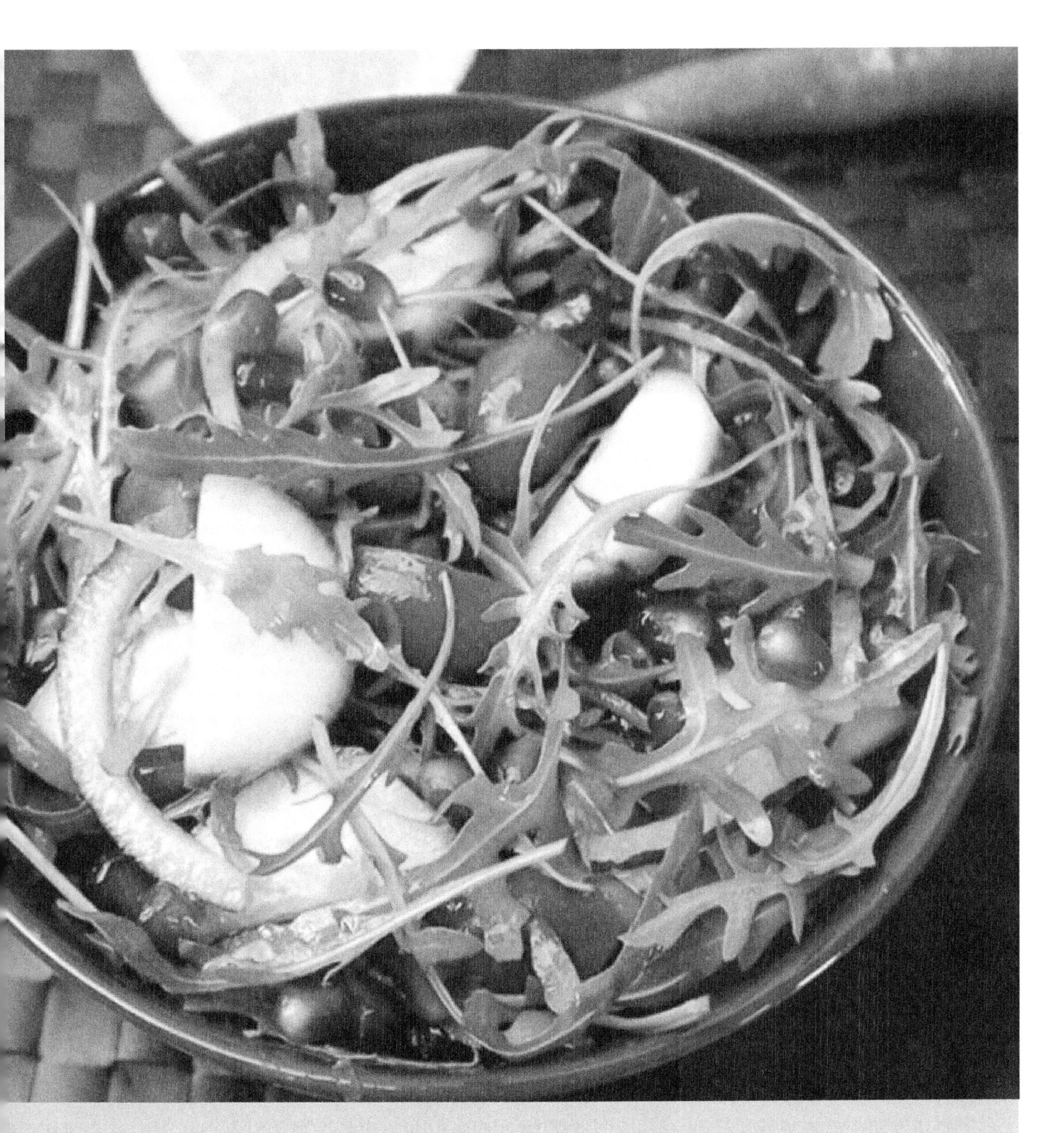

Chapter 7:
Salad

Easy Kale Salad with Fresh Lemon Dressing

PREP TIME: 20 minutes Serves: 4
TOTAL TIME: 20 minutes

10

This easy kale salad features fresh veggies and a super simple homemade lemon dressing, making it perfect as a healthy side dish or light lunch!

- 5 cups kale chopped
- 1-2 teaspoons olive oil
- ⅛ teaspoon salt
- 2 cups broccoli chopped
- ½ cup almonds sliced
- ½ cup cheese optional (cheddar or feta work great here!)
- ¼-½ cup carrots shredded
- ¼ cup red onion diced
- ¼ cup sunflower seeds
- ¼ cup cranberries

Lemon Dressing
- ¼ cup olive oil
- 2 tablespoons fresh lemon juice
- 2 tablespoons red wine vinegar
- 1 tablespoon dijon mustard
- 1 clove garlic minced
- ½ teaspoon dried oregano
- ¼ teaspoon salt
- ⅛ teaspoon ground black pepper
- 1 teaspoon honey or sugar adjust + add to taste

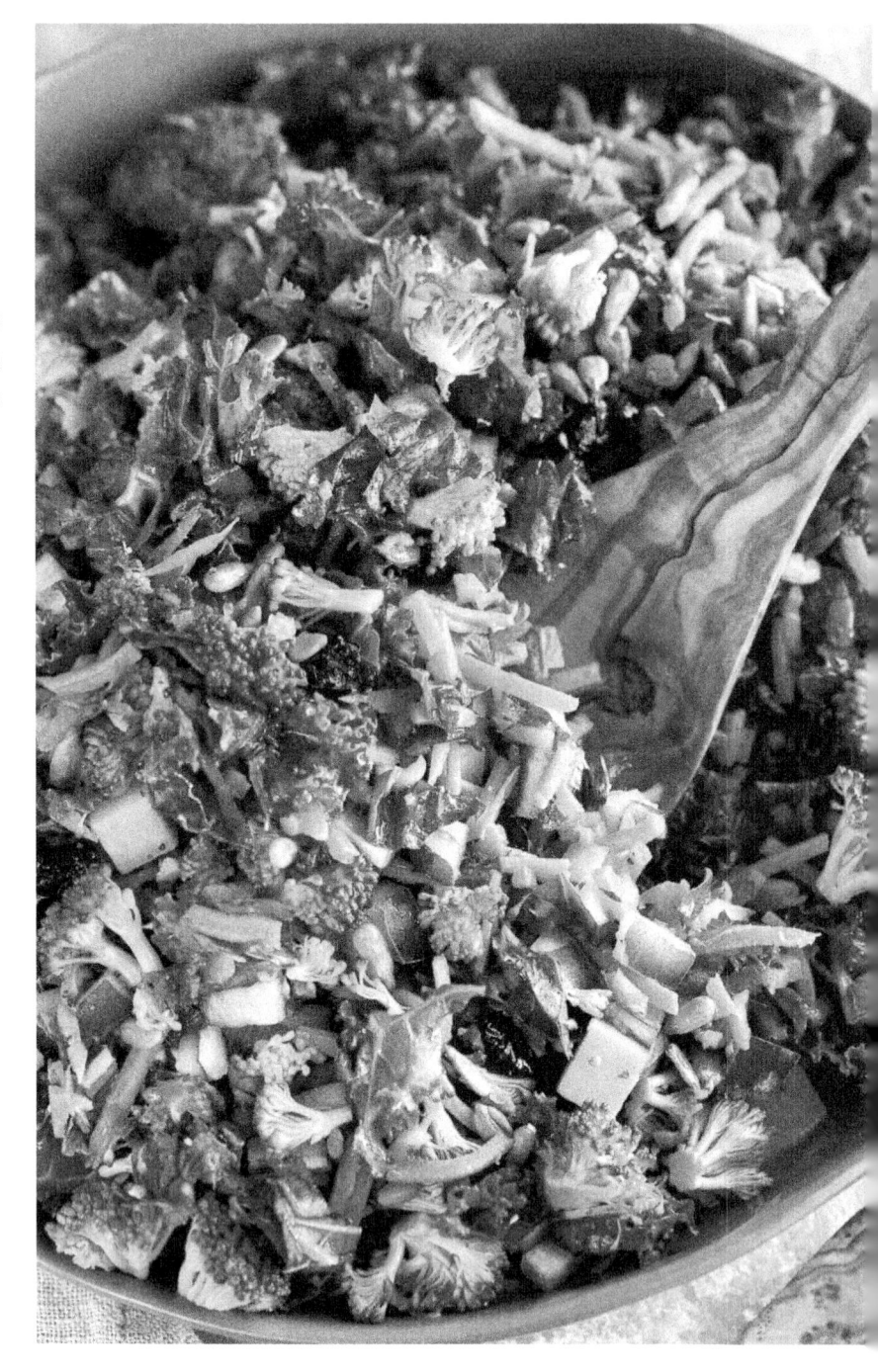

1. First make your dressing by combining ingredients above in a lidded mason jar then shake well to emulsify. Dip a kale leaf in the dressing and adjust sweetener, salt, and pepper to taste. You can make this dressing as sweet or tart as your heart desires!
2. Next massage your chopped kale with a little olive oil and a pinch of salt. Rub with your fingers until leaves begin to darken and tenderize. This makes it taste great and gives the kale a silky texture!
3. In a large bowl, combine massaged kale, broccoli, almonds, cheese, carrots, onion, sunflower seeds, cranberries. Shake your dressing once more and pour about ⅓ of the dressing over the salad. Toss to coat and add extra dressing, to taste.

NUTRITION FACTS

Calories: 334, Carbohydrates: 19g, Protein: 9g, Fat: 26g, Saturated Fat: 3g, Sodium: 315mg, Potassium: 744mg, Fiber: 4g, Sugar: 4g, Vitamin A: 9985IU, Vitamin C: 146.3mg, Calcium: 192mg, Iron: 2.7mg

The Best Coleslaw Recipe

PREP TIME: 20 minutes Serves: 6
CHILL TIME: 1 hour
TOTAL TIME: 1 hour 20 minutes

5

This creamy coleslaw is the best salad or sandwich topper. It's the perfect make-ahead dish, ideal for a BBQ or potluck!

- 3 cups green cabbage finely shredded
- 2 cups purple cabbage finely shredded
- 1 cup carrot finely shredded

Dressing
- ½ cup mayonnaise/dressing
- 1 tablespoon white vinegar
- ½ tablespoon cider vinegar
- 2 teaspoons sugar
- ½ teaspoon celery seeds
- salt & pepper to taste

1. Combine all dressing ingredients in a bowl.
2. Toss with cabbage & carrots. Refrigerate at least 1 hour before serving to allow flavors to blend.

Recipe Notes
1. Cabbage and carrots above can be replaced with coleslaw mix.
2. Don't skip the celery seed, it really adds a lot of flavor to this dish.
3. This dish is best after the flavors have had a chance to blend. Resting in the fridge also helps to soften the slaw.

Option 2: Vinaigrette Coleslaw Dressing:
- 3 tablespoons apple cider vinegar
- 4 tablespoons canola oil
- 3 tablespoons white sugar
- ½ teaspoon dijon mustard
- ¼ teaspoon celery seeds
- salt & pepper to taste

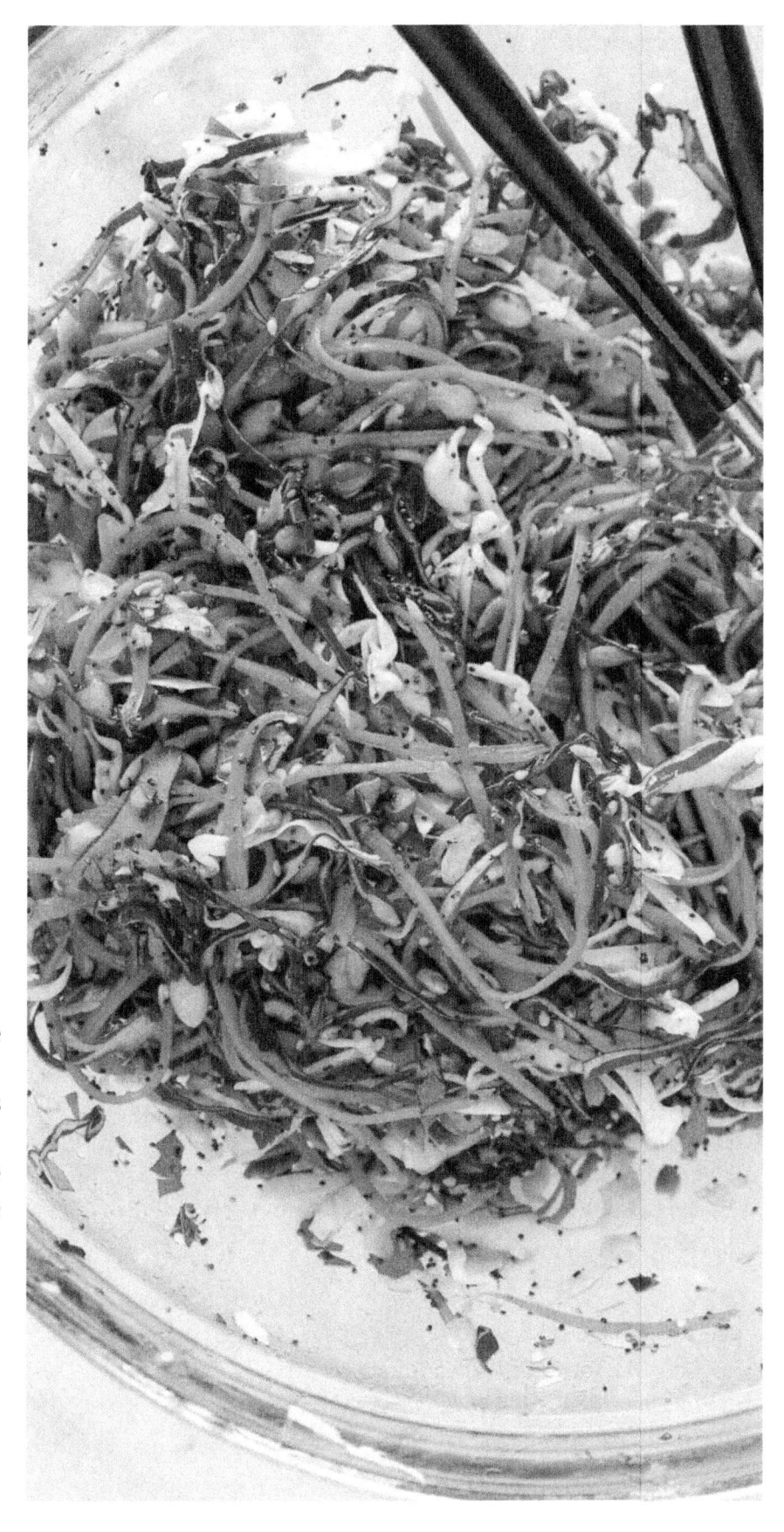

NUTRITION FACTS

Calories: 160, Carbohydrates: 8g, Protein: 1g, Fat: 14g, Saturated Fat: 2g, Polyunsaturated Fat: 8g, Monounsaturated Fat: 3g, Trans Fat: 1g, Cholesterol: 8mg, Sodium: 148mg, Potassium: 207mg, Fiber: 2g, Sugar: 5g, Vitamin A: 3942IU, Vitamin C: 31mg, Calcium: 39mg, Iron: 1mg

Chickpea Salad

PREP TIME: 20 minutes
COOK TIME: 0 minutes
TOTAL TIME: 20 minutes

Serves: 6

5

This beautiful Chickpea Salad combines all of my favorite fresh vegetables in one delicious bite. Chickpeas are combined with juicy tomatoes, refreshing cucumbers, and creamy avocados all tossed in an easy homemade lemon kissed dressing.

- 1 avocado
- ½ fresh lemon
- 2 cups grape tomatoes sliced
- 2 cups cucumber diced
- 1 can chickpeas drained (19 ounces)
- ¾ cup green bell pepper diced
- ½ cup fresh parsley chopped
- ¼ cup red onion sliced

Dressing
- ¼ cup olive oil
- 2 tablespoons red wine vinegar
- ½ teaspoon cumin
- salt & pepper

1. Cut avocado into cubes and place in a bowl. Squeeze the juice from the lemon over the avocado and gently stir to combine.
2. Add remaining salad ingredients and gently toss to combine.
3. Refrigerate at least one hour before serving.

Recipe Notes
- Store leftover Chickpea Salad covered in the fridge for up to 3 days. Stir to refresh flavors and serve cold.

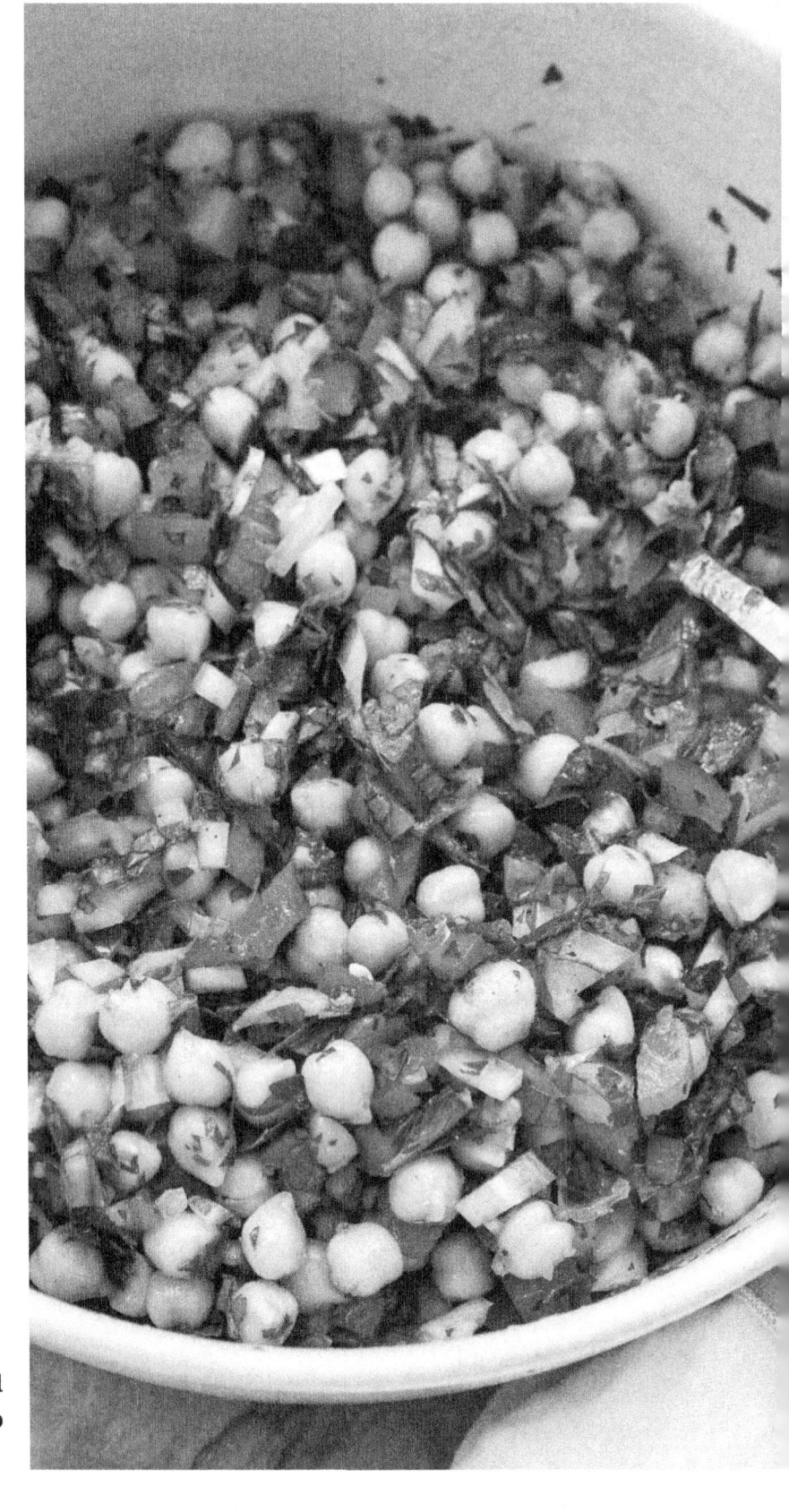

NUTRITION FACTS

Calories: 238, Carbohydrates: 20g, Protein: 6g, Fat: 15g, Saturated Fat: 2g, Sodium: 259mg, Potassium: 552mg, Fiber: 7g, Sugar: 3g, Vitamin A: 1000IU, Vitamin C: 38.4mg, Calcium: 58mg, Iron: 2.1mg

Easy Pasta Salad Recipe

PREP TIME: 20 minutes Serves: 8
COOK TIME: 15 minutes
CHILL TIME: 2 hours
TOTAL TIME: 2 hours 35 minutes

`10`

Pasta Salad with fresh veggies, ham, and a tangy Italian dressing is perfect for a potluck or backyard BBQ!

- 1 pound medium pasta such as rotini, farfalle or penne
- 1 cup mozzarella cheese cubed
- 1 cup chopped ham or salami
- 1 english cucumber chopped
- 1 pint grape tomatoes halved
- 1 bell pepper chopped
- ¼ cup black olives sliced, or to taste
- 4 green onions thinly sliced
- 1 cup Italian dressing homemade or store-bought, or your favorite dressing
- 3 tablespoons fresh parsley chopped
- salt & pepper to taste

1. Cook pasta al dente according to package directions. Rinse under cold water.
2. While pasta is cooking, prepare vegetables.
3. Place all ingredients in a large bowl and mix well.
4. Refrigerate at least 2 hours before serving.

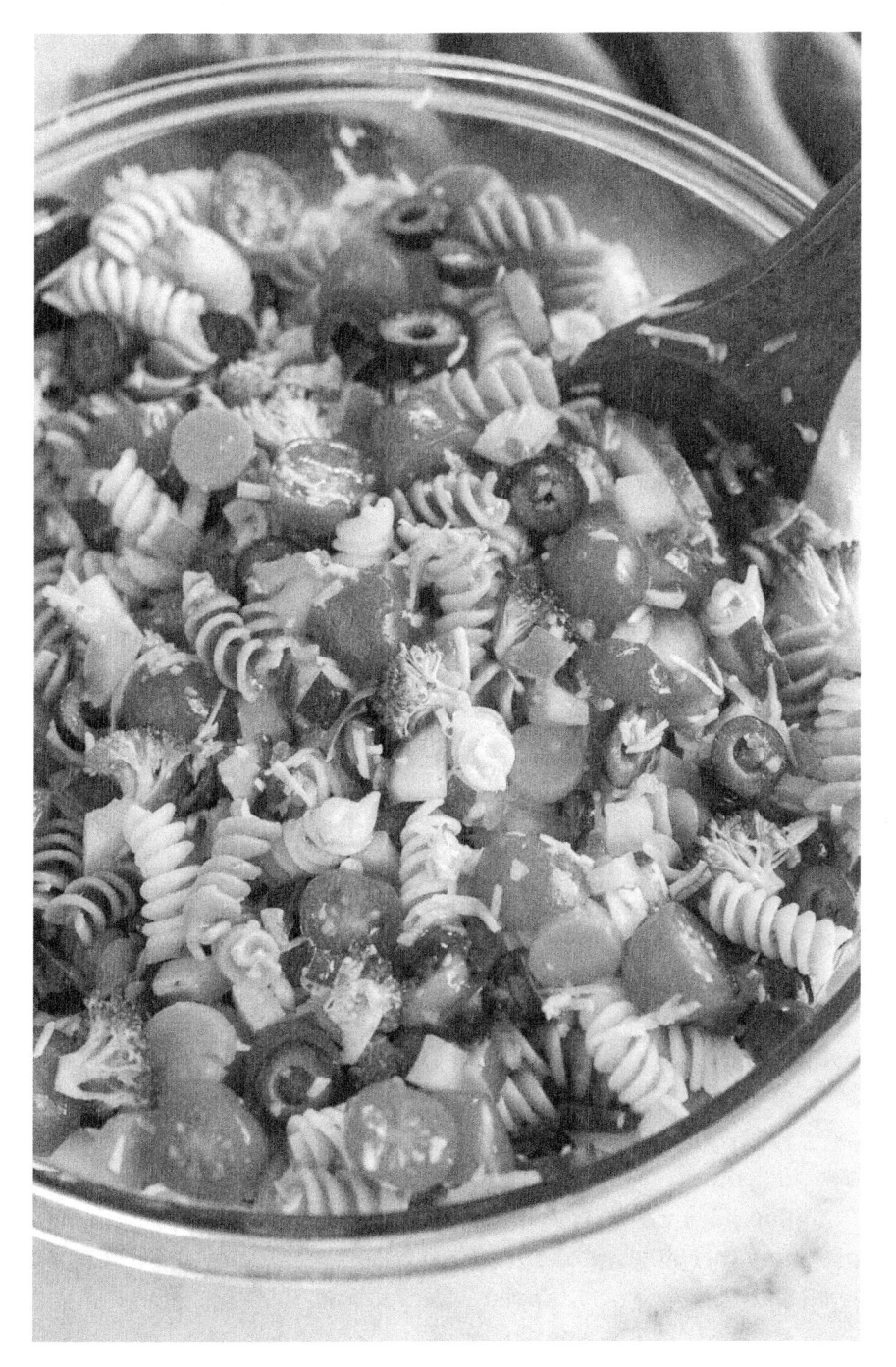

Recipe Notes

- Any medium pasta can be used. Be sure to cook al dente (firm) as the dressing will soften the pasta further. Rinse under cold water once cooked to stop it from cooking.
- You can use any vegetables in this recipe (including leftover cooked/roasted vegetables). Favorites include zucchini, peas, peppers, tomatoes, and cucumbers.
- Optional but delicious additions include bacon, sundried tomatoes, pesto, artichokes, or finely diced broccoli.
- Dress the salad generously as the pasta will soak up the dressing.

NUTRITION FACTS

Serving: 1.5cup, Calories: 303, Carbohydrates: 36g, Protein: 10g, Fat: 13g, Saturated Fat: 3g, Trans Fat: 1g, Cholesterol: 15mg, Sodium: 579mg, Potassium: 324mg, Fiber: 2g, Sugar: 7g, Vitamin A: 866IU, Vitamin C: 21mg, Calcium: 74mg, Iron: 1mg

Creamy Cranberry Salad

PREP TIME: 15 minutes
COOK TIME: 45 minutes
CHILL TIME: 2 hours
TOTAL TIME: 3 hours

Serves: 6

13

Deliciously sweet and tart, this Cranberry Jello Salad is perfect for any occasion. It's festive, colorful, and tasty!

- 12 ounces cranberries fresh or frozen
- ½ cup sugar
- ¼ cup orange juice
- 1 tablespoon lemon juice
- 1 package raspberry Jello 3 ounces or 85g
- 1 cup heavy whipping cream
- 2 tablespoons powdered sugar

1. Bring cranberries, sugar, orange juice, and lemon juice to a boil. Simmer 7-8 minutes or until the cranberries pop and are cooked. Remove from heat and stir in Jello. Cool completely.
2. Combine heavy cream and powdered sugar in a bowl. Whip until stiff peaks form.
3. Fold the cream into the cranberry mixture.
4. Spread into a bowl and refrigerate until set, at least 2 hours or overnight.
5. Garnish with whipped cream and sugared cranberries if desired.

Recipe Notes
- To store leftovers, cover with plastic wrap in the fridge for up to 3 days.

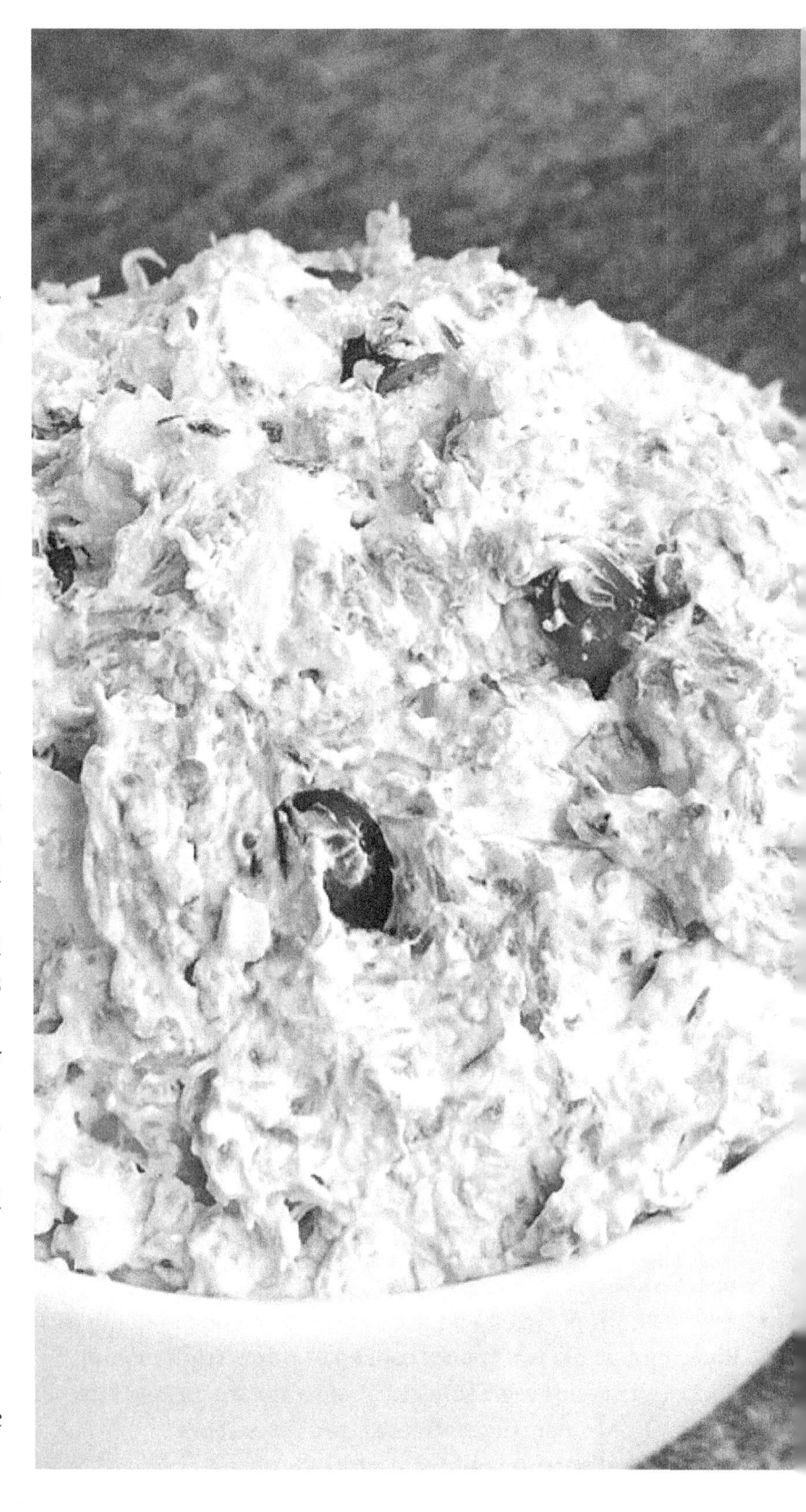

NUTRITION FACTS

Calories: 297, Carbohydrates: 41g, Protein: 2g, Fat: 15g, Saturated Fat: 9g, Polyunsaturated Fat: 1g, Monounsaturated Fat: 4g, Cholesterol: 54mg, Sodium: 83mg, Potassium: 103mg, Fiber: 3g, Sugar: 35g, Vitamin A: 638IU, Vitamin C: 14mg, Calcium: 32mg, Iron: 1mg

Old Fashioned Three Bean Salad

PREP TIME: 15 minutes   Serves: 12
COOK TIME: 10 minutes
CHILL TIME: 12 hours
TOTAL TIME: 12 hours 25 minutes

4

This Bean Salad has been a family staple for years. 4 kinds of beans and a hint of white onion, all dressed in a sweet tangy vinaigrette dressing.

- 14 ounces green beans
- 14 ounces yellow beans
- 14 ounces red kidney beans
- 14 ounces lima beans optional
- ½ cup green pepper thinly sliced
- ¾ cup white onion thinly sliced
- ¾ cup celery chopped

DRESSING

- ⅔ cup white sugar
- ½ cup white vinegar
- ½ cup vegetable oil
- 1 teaspoon salt
- 1 teaspoon celery seeds
- ½ teaspoon pepper

1. Drain all of the beans well. Combine beans, green pepper, celery and onion in a bowl.
2. Heat all dressing ingredients in a small saucepan until sugar is dissolved and mixture is hot.
3. Pour the hot dressing mixture over the beans and toss to coat. Refrigerate overnight turning or stirring occasionally.

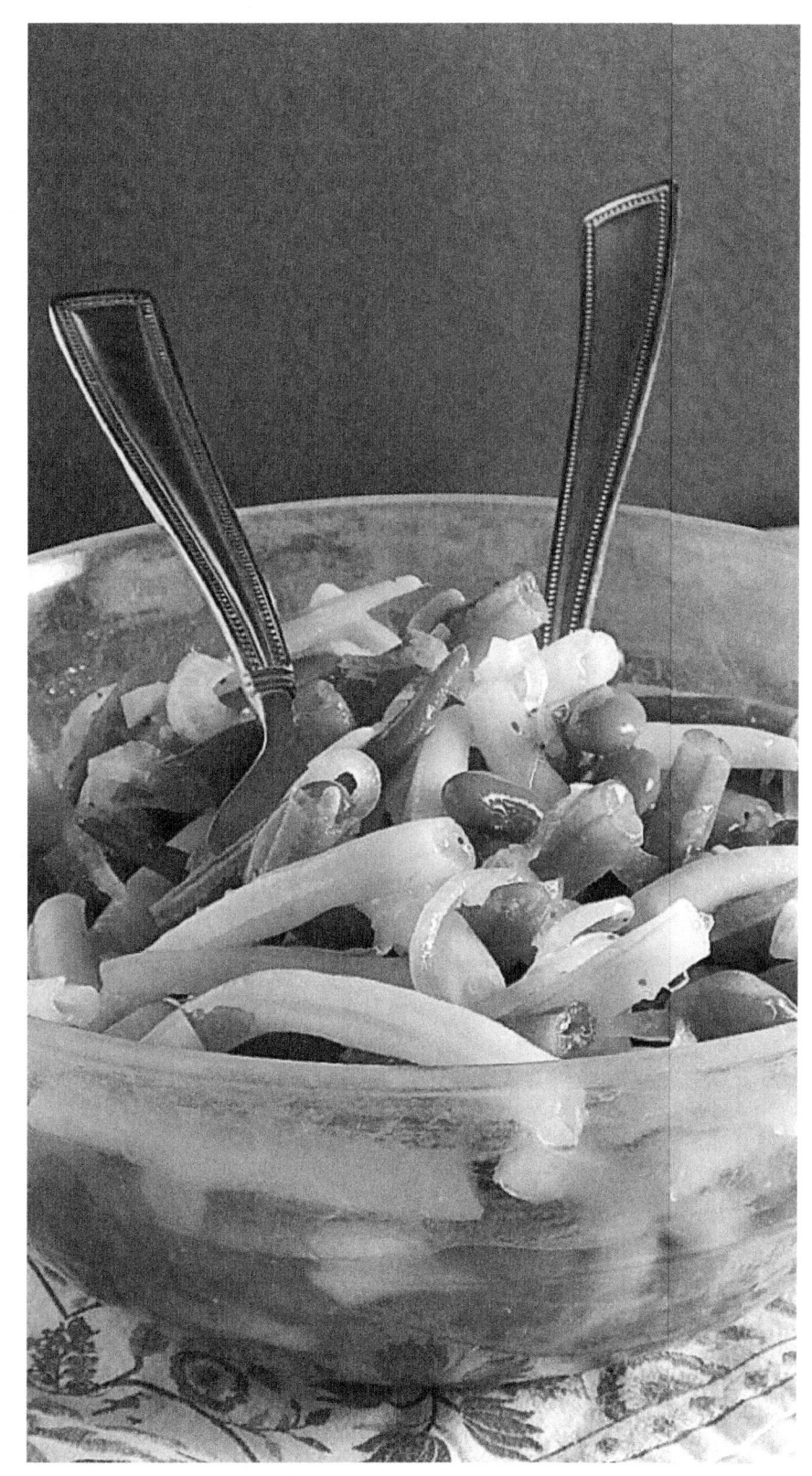

NUTRITION FACTS

Calories: 154, Carbohydrates: 32g, Protein: 7g, Fat: 1g, Saturated Fat: 1g, Polyunsaturated Fat: 1g, Monounsaturated Fat: 1g, Sodium: 205mg, Potassium: 486mg, Fiber: 7g, Sugar: 14g, Vitamin A: 280IU, Vitamin C: 17mg, Calcium: 52mg, Iron: 3mg

Brussels Sprout Salad

PREP TIME: 20 minutes Serves: 6
COOK TIME: 10 minutes
TOTAL TIME: 30 minutes

8

Shredded Brussels sprouts, crisp tart apples, feta cheese, cranberries, pomegranate arils, and walnuts all tossed in a tangy honey dijon vinaigrette.

- 1 ½ pounds fresh Brussels sprouts shredded
- 1 apple granny smith , or any variety
- 1 teaspoon lemon juice
- ⅓ cup dried cranberries or dried cherries
- ⅓ cup pomegranate arils
- ¼ cup walnuts or pecans, chopped
- 2 ounces feta cheese crumbled

Dressing
- ⅓ cup olive oil
- 3 tablespoons cider vinegar
- 1 tablespoon fresh lemon juice
- 2 tablespoons honey
- 1 ½ teaspoons dijon mustard
- ½ teaspoon garlic powder
- salt and pepper to taste

1. Combine all dressing ingredients in a small jar and shake well to combine.
2. Shred Brussels sprouts, rinse well and dry.
3. Chop apple and toss with lemon juice to prevent browning.
4. Combine all remaining salad ingredients in a large salad bowl. Toss with dressing and serve.

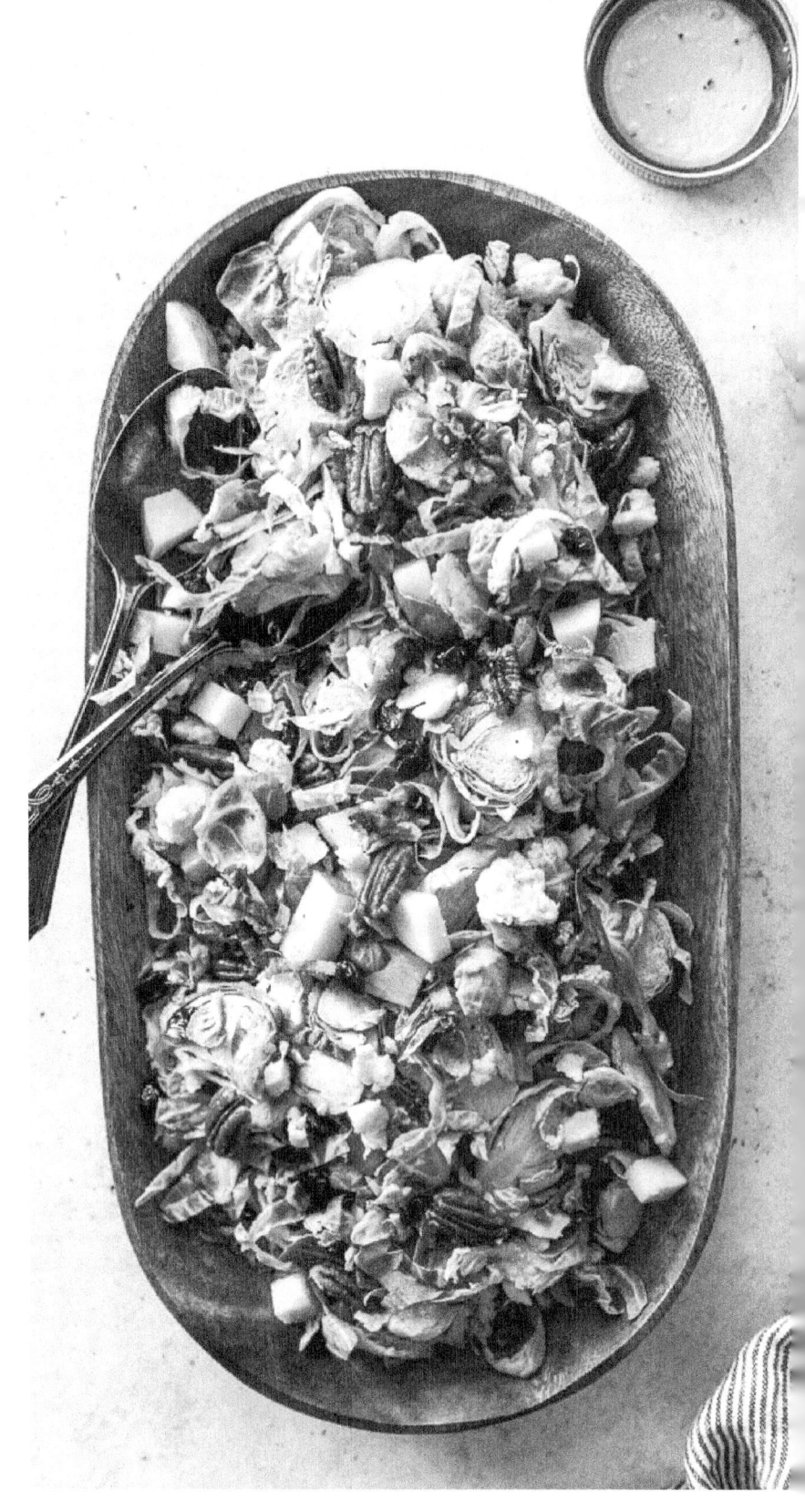

NUTRITION FACTS

Calories: 281, Carbohydrates: 28g, Protein: 6g, Fat: 17g, Saturated Fat: 3g, Cholesterol: 8mg, Sodium: 149mg, Potassium: 516mg, Fiber: 6g, Sugar: 17g, Vitamin A: 910IU, Vitamin C: 100mg, Calcium: 101mg, Iron: 1.9mg

Avocado Corn Salad

PREP TIME: 20 minutes **Serves:** 4
COOK TIME: 5 minutes
TOTAL TIME: 25 minutes

`10`

Avocado Corn Salad is a fresh and colorful salad that goes perfect with any meal!

- 2 cups corn or 2 cobs fresh corn
- ½ teaspoon cumin
- 2 tablespoons olive oil + 1 teaspoon
- 1 ½ cups grape tomatoes halved
- 2 ripe avocados
- 1 lime juiced
- 1 green onion chopped
- ¼ cup fresh cilantro or parsley, chopped
- 2 tablespoons feta cheese
- 1 tablespoon white wine vinegar
- 1 clove garlic minced
- salt & pepper to taste
- 8 cups spring mix

1. Toss corn with cumin and salt & pepper to taste. Heat a skillet over medium high heat and add 1 teaspoon oil and corn. Cook 5-7 minutes or until corn begins to brown. Cool completely.
2. Cut avocados in half, remove pits, and dice. Squeeze fresh lime juice over avocados and gently toss to combine.
3. Add remaining ingredients (except for lettuce) with the cooled corn and avocado to a bowl and gently stir to combine.
4. Let stand 5-10 minutes.
5. Divide lettuce over bowls and top with corn mixture.
6. Optional additions: cheese, bell peppers, cucumbers

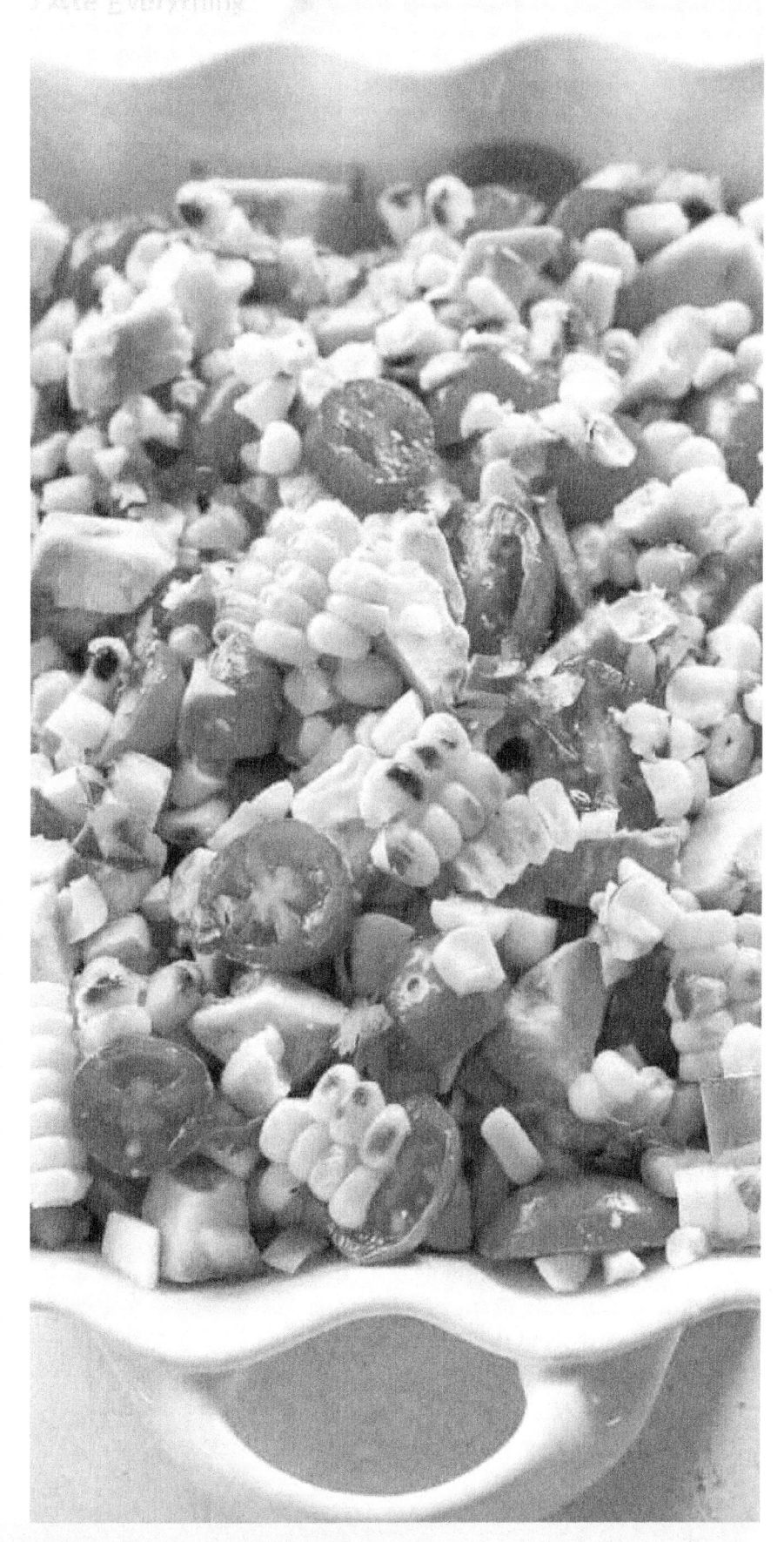

NUTRITION FACTS

Calories: 351, Carbohydrates: 32g, Protein: 8g, Fat: 25g, Saturated Fat: 5g, Polyunsaturated Fat: 3g, Monounsaturated Fat: 16g, Cholesterol: 8mg, Sodium: 129mg, Potassium: 970mg, Fiber: 10g, Sugar: 6g, Vitamin A: 1868IU, Vitamin C: 46mg, Calcium: 85mg, Iron: 2mg

Easy Arugula Salad

PREP TIME: 15 minutes   Serves: 4
COOK TIME: 10 minutes
TOTAL TIME: 25 minutes

10

Fresh, crisp, and totally flavorful, this easy arugula salad is perfect for a light lunch or dinner!

- 6 cups arugula washed & dried
- 1 cup cherry tomatoes
- 1 ounce parmesan petals see notes
- ¼ cup red onion finely sliced
- 1 tablespoon toasted pine nuts or toasted almonds

Lemon Vinaigrette
- ¼ cup vegetable oil
- 1 ½ tablespoon red wine vinegar
- 1 tablespoon fresh lemon juice
- 1 teaspoon dijon mustard
- ½ teaspoon sugar or to taste

1. Whisk all dressing ingredients except the oil in a medium bowl.
2. Slowly drizzle oil into the mixture while whisking. Season to taste with salt & pepper.
3. Place arugula in a large salad bowl and toss with dressing. Add remaining ingredients on top.
4. Serve immediately.

Recipe Notes
1. Parmesan petals can be made by shaving pieces off the block of Parmesan with a vegetable peeler.
2. Add spinach in place of some of the arugula to soften the flavor.
3. Substitute store bought dressings for homemade. Choose dressings with a sweet tangy flavor like honey mustard or poppy seed.

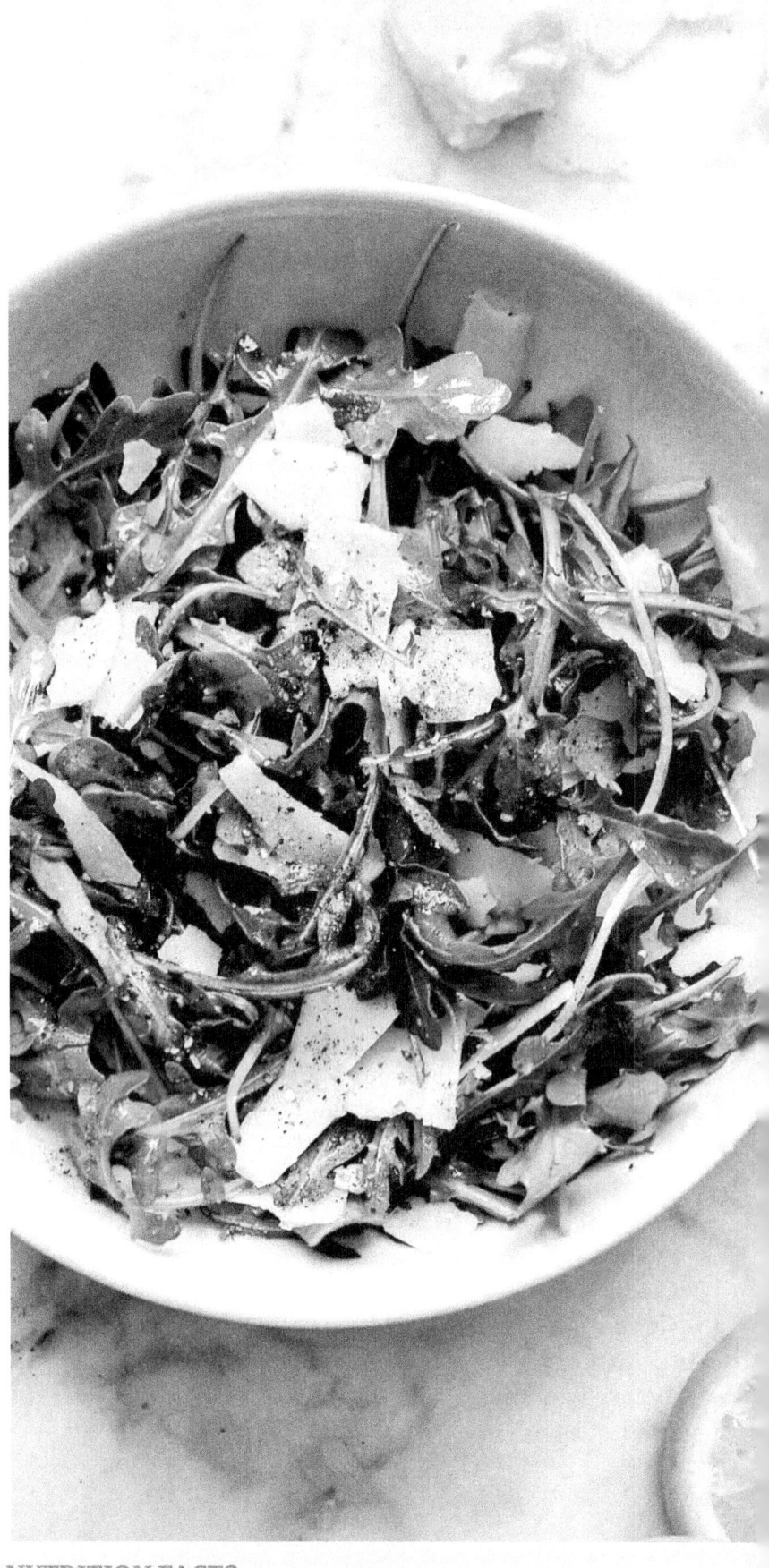

NUTRITION FACTS

Calories: 185, Carbohydrates: 5g, Protein: 4g, Fat: 17g, Saturated Fat: 12g, Polyunsaturated Fat: 1g, Monounsaturated Fat: 3g, Cholesterol: 5mg, Sodium: 141mg, Potassium: 236mg, Fiber: 1g, Sugar: 3g, Vitamin A: 951IU, Vitamin C: 15mg, Calcium: 140mg, Iron: 1mg

Easy Taco Salad

PREP TIME: 15 minutes **Serves:** 8
COOK TIME: 15 minutes
TOTAL TIME: 30 minutes

11

This easy taco salad is crispy, crunchy and colorful! It is so much fun to put together because you can customize the toppings, making everyone at the dinner table happy!

Beef
- 1 pound lean ground beef
- 1 package taco seasoning or homemade
- 1 cup black beans drained and rinsed

Salad
- 6 cups romaine or iceberg lettuce, chopped
- 1 cup tomatoes chopped
- 1 cup cheddar cheese shredded
- 1 avocado diced
- 1 cup tortilla chips
- ½ cup salsa
- ½ cup sour cream
- toppings as desired olives, bell peppers, jalapenos, red or green onion

1. Brown beef over medium heat until no pink remains. Drain any fat.
2. Add taco seasoning and ½ cup water. Simmer 5 minutes or until thickened. Stir in beans.
3. Place lettuce in a large bowl. Top with meat, tomatoes, cheese, avocado and desired toppings.
4. Top each serving with tortilla chips, salsa and sour cream.

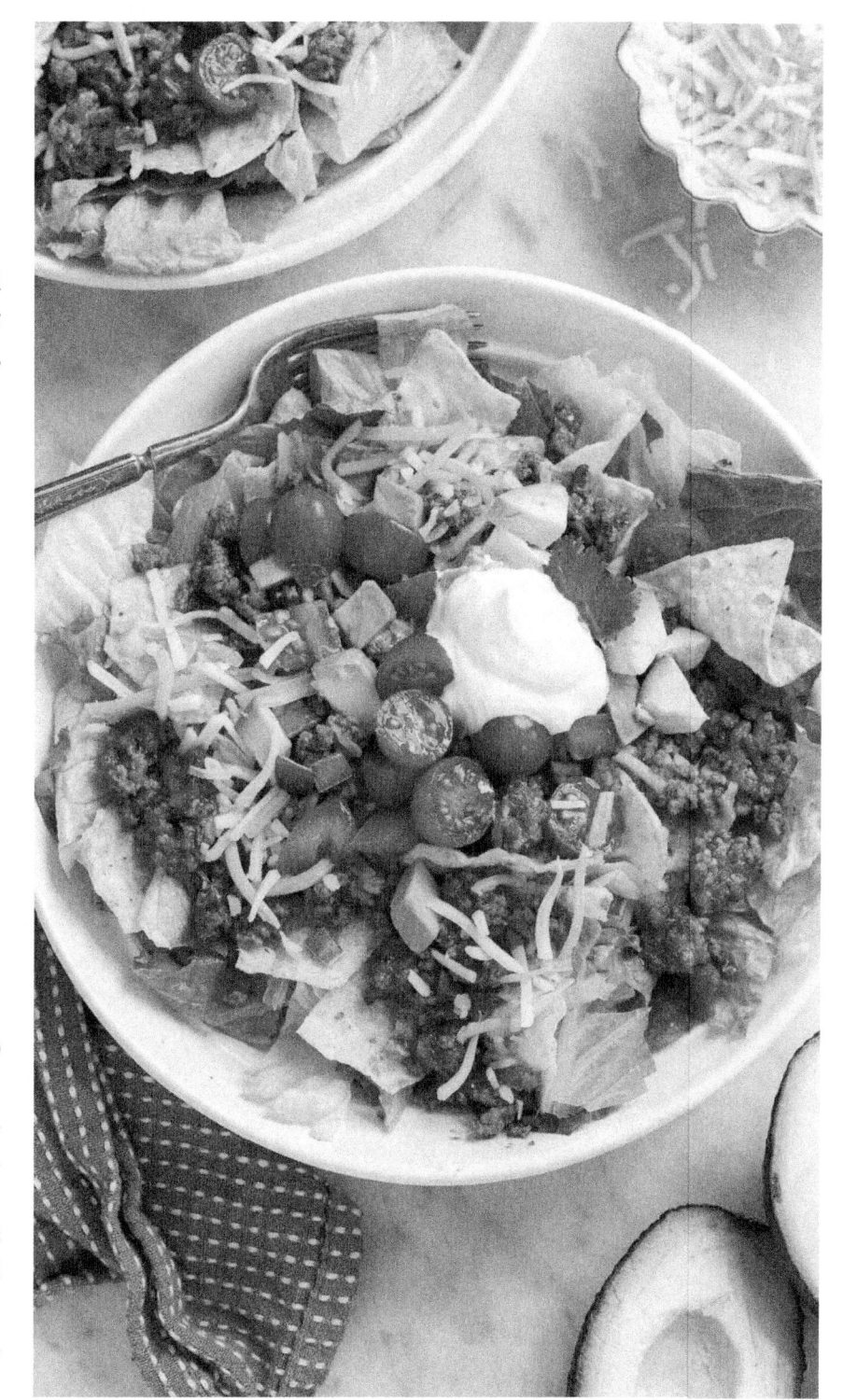

Recipe Notes
1. While we use sour cream and salsa as dressing, catalina or Thousand Island are also great tossed with this salad.
2. To make this meal fast, use pre-washed lettuce. Prepare topping ingredients while the meat is cooking.

NUTRITION FACTS

Calories: 360, Carbohydrates: 20g, Protein: 19g, Fat: 23g, Saturated Fat: 9g, Cholesterol: 61mg, Sodium: 328mg, Potassium: 608mg, Fiber: 6g, Sugar: 2g, Vitamin A: 3585IU, Vitamin C: 6.9mg, Calcium: 178mg, Iron: 2.7mg

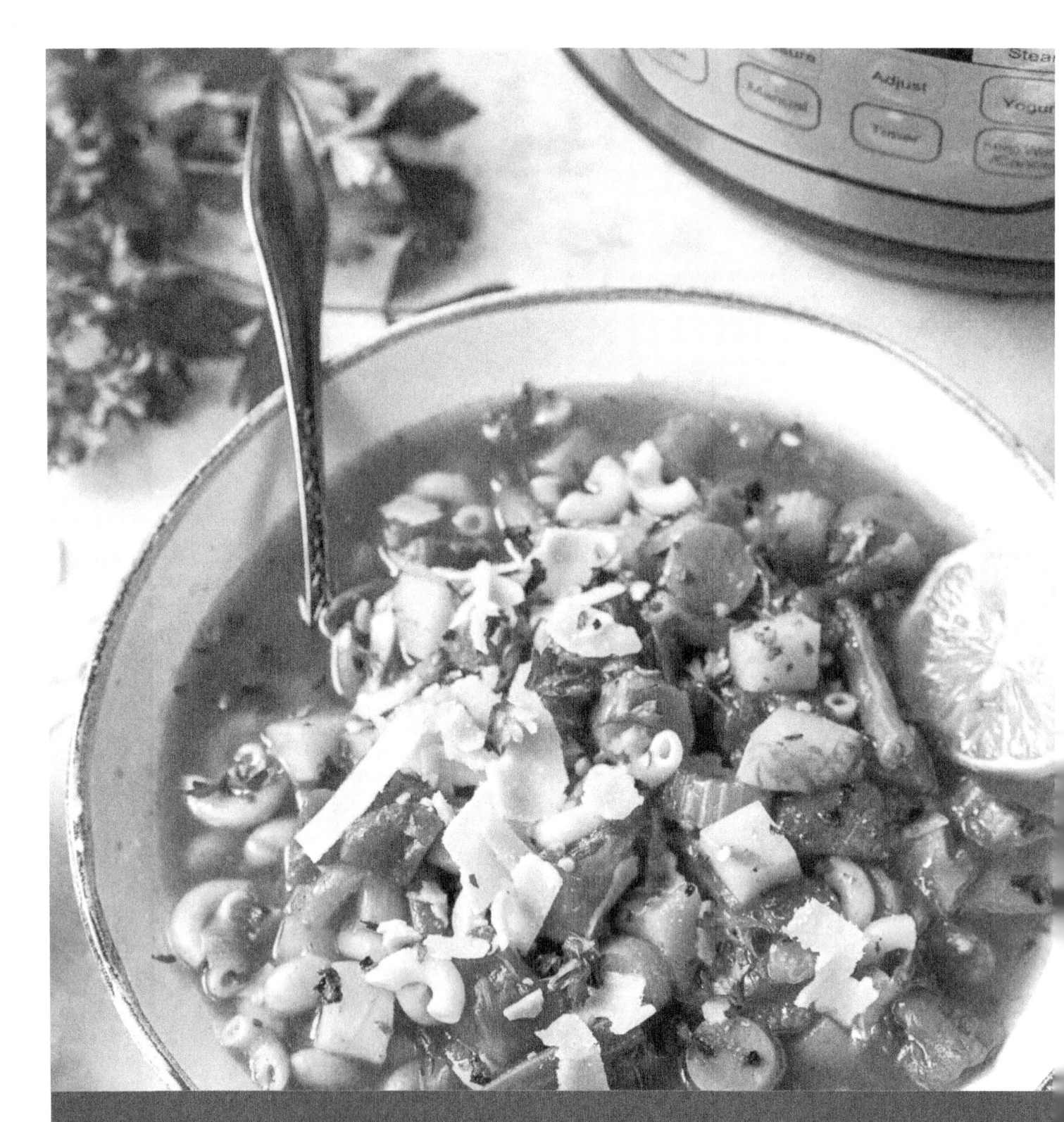

Chapter 8:
Instant Pot

Instant Pot Minestrone Soup

PREP TIME: 20 minutes   Serves: 6
COOK TIME: 20 minutes
TOTAL TIME: 40 minutes

7

We love this easy Minestrone Soup loaded with healthy, colorful veggies and cooked in the Instant Pot!

- 1 tablespoon oil vegetable or olive
- 1 onion finely diced
- 3 large carrots chopped
- 2 ribs celery sliced
- 6 cups low sodium chicken broth
- 28 ounces canned diced tomatoes with juice
- 15.5 ounces canned red kidney beans drained and rinsed
- 15.5 ounces canned cannellini beans drained and rinsed
- 1 ½ cups mini shell pasta uncooked
- ½ zucchini sliced into ½" half moons
- 2 cloves garlic minced
- 1 ½ teaspoons salt
- 1 ½ teaspoons dried Italian seasoning
- 2 bay leaves
- ⅛ teaspoon black pepper
- 2 cups fresh spinach chopped
- fresh basil, parsley, and/or parmesan cheese for serving optional

1. Turn a 6 qt Instant Pot onto SAUTÉ.
2. Once heated, add oil, onion, carrots, and celery. Cook while stirring until the onions are slightly softened, about 3 minutes.
3. Add broth and use a spatula to scrape up any brown bits in the bottom of the Instant Pot.
4. Add remaining ingredients except for the spinach & basil if using.
5. Put the lid on the Instant Pot and set it to MANUAL (or PRESSURE COOK) on HIGH pressure for 4 minutes.
6. When the cooking time is done, quick release the pressure and open the lid. Stir in spinach and let rest 5-10 minutes.
7. Remove the bay leaves and discard.
8. Serve with shredded parmesan cheese and fresh basil or parsley if desired.

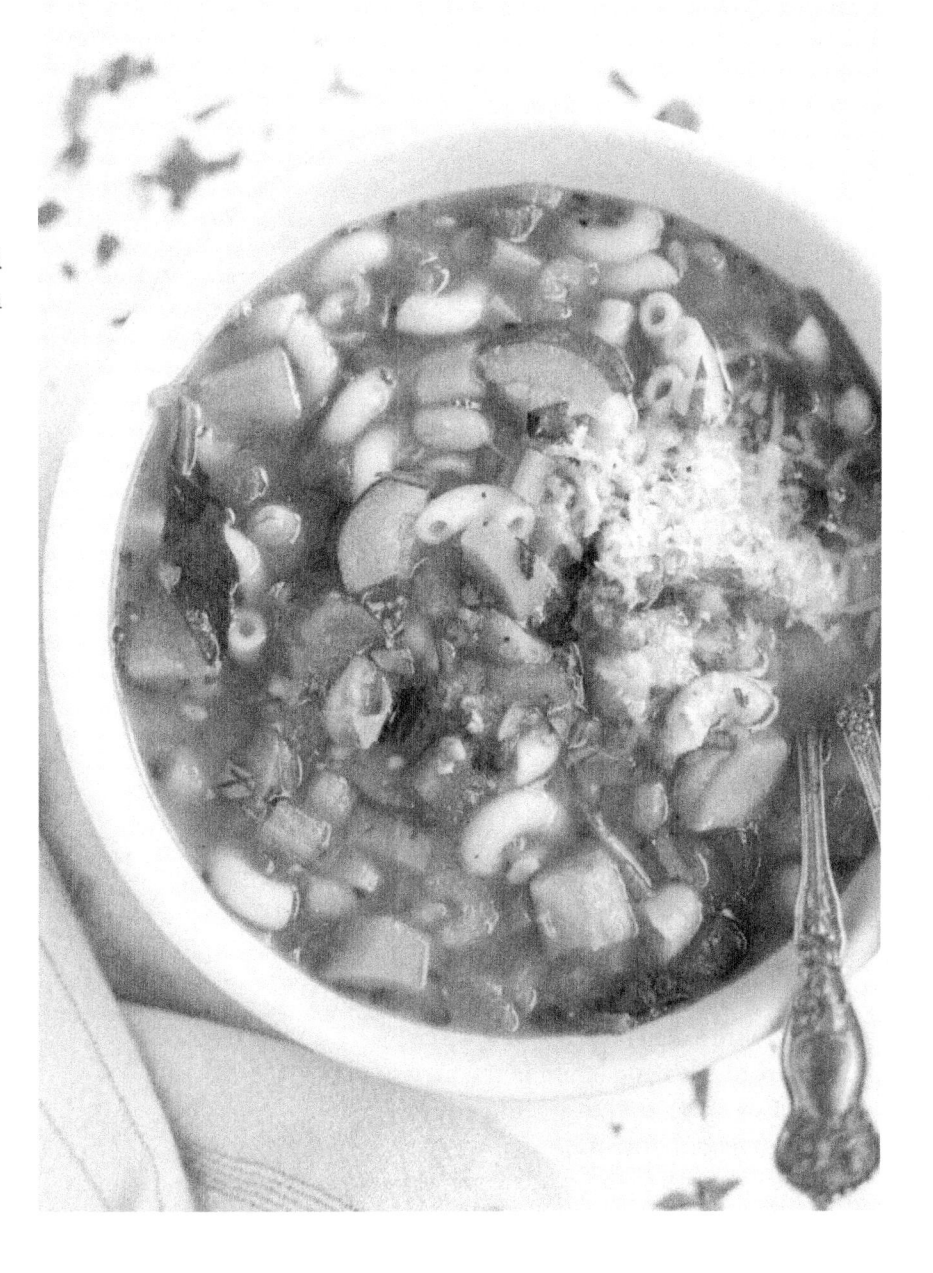

NUTRITION FACTS

Calories: 349, Carbohydrates: 60g, Protein: 19g, Fat: 5g, Saturated Fat: 1g, Polyunsaturated Fat: 2g, Monounsaturated Fat: 2g, Trans Fat: 1g, Sodium: 1080mg, Potassium: 1317mg, Fiber: 12g, Sugar: 9g, Vitamin A: 7210IU, Vitamin C: 23mg, Calcium: 175mg, Iron: 6mg

Instant Pot Corned Beef

PREP TIME: 20 minutes   Serves: 6
COOK TIME: 1 hour 30 minutes
TOTAL TIME: 1 hour 50 minutes

This recipe makes for a hearty entrée all year round, especially on those chilly winter days!

- 2 cups water or broth
- 6 ounces beer
- 6 ounces beef broth
- 1 large onion chopped
- 4 cloves garlic minced
- 2-3 pound corned beef brisket with spice packet
- 1 pound baby potatoes
- 3 cups cabbage chopped
- 3 carrots chopped

1. Combine water, beer, broth, onion, and garlic in a 6QT Instant Pot.
2. Add the trivet and add the corned beef brisket with the *spice mixture (if yours doesn't have a spice mixture, see note).
3. Cook on high pressure for 90 minutes. Once done, release pressure and remove brisket, tent with foil to rest.
4. Leave about 1 cup liquid in the Instant Pot. Add cabbage, potatoes and carrots. Set to high pressure for 5 minutes.
5. Quick-release pressure. Remove vegetables to a serving plate with a slotted spoon. Top with butter or sauce from the Instant Pot.
6. Slice corned beef across the grain and serve with vegetables.

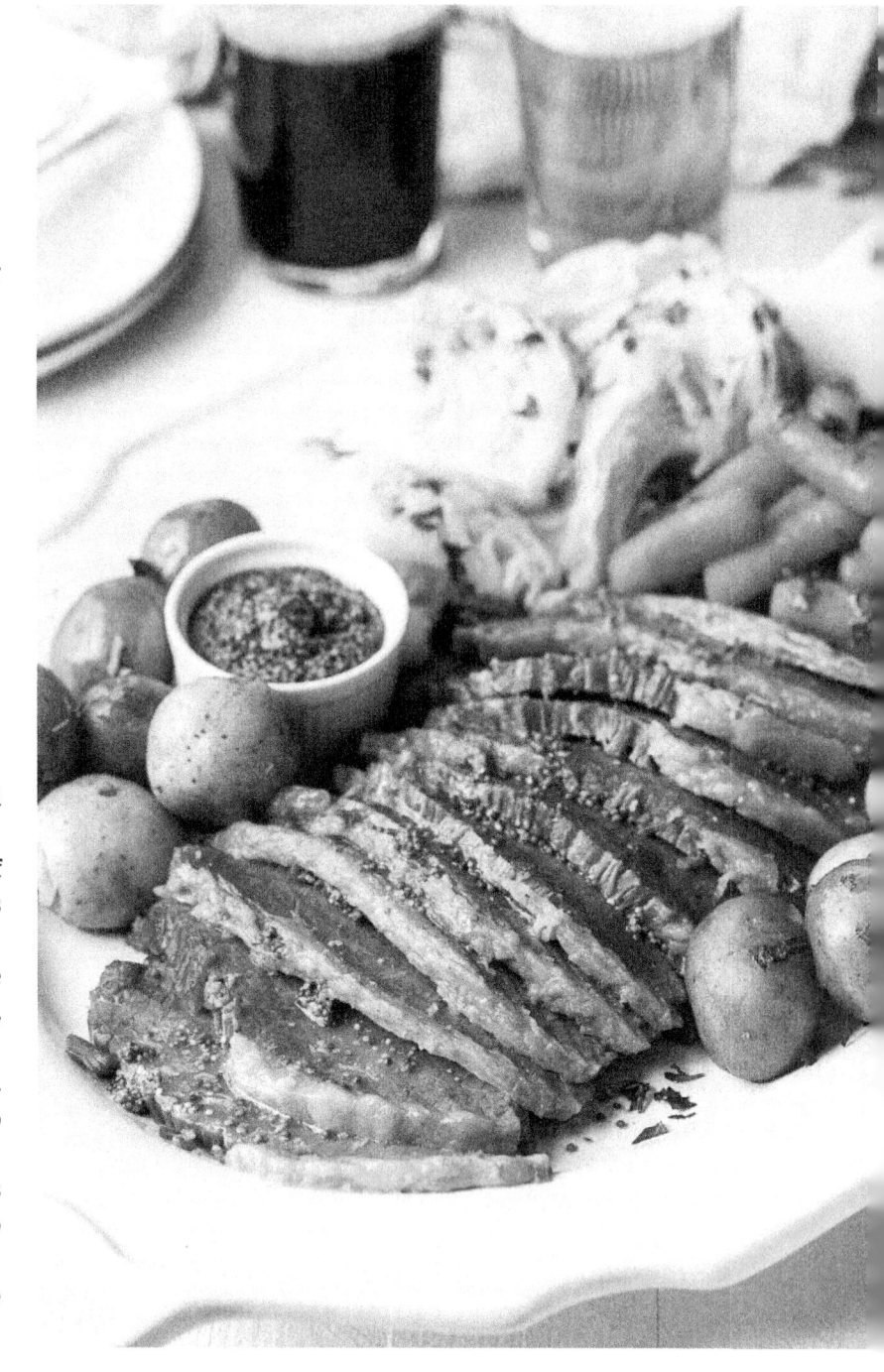

Recipe Notes
1. Corned beef often comes with a spice packet to be added during cooking. If you don't see a spice packet, sometimes the spices are already in the beef and the packet is not separate. A corned beef spice packet can be substituted with about tablespoon or so of pickling spices.
2. You can use all broth or all beer with the water. Darker beers can produce a slightly bitter flavor depending on the type/brand.
3. I prefer baby potatoes because they hold their shape and don't require peeling/chopping but you can use any potatoes. Russet potatoes will need to be peeled. Baby carrots will work in this recipe.

NUTRITION FACTS

Calories: 416, Carbohydrates: 23g, Protein: 25g, Fat: 23g, Saturated Fat: 7g, Cholesterol: 82mg, Sodium: 1880mg, Potassium: 984mg, Fiber: 4g, Sugar: 4g, Vitamin A: 5130IU, Vitamin C: 73mg, Calcium: 58mg, Iron: 3mg

Instant Pot Spaghetti

PREP TIME: 20 minutes   Serves: 6
COOK TIME: 8 minutes
BUILDING PRESSURE & RESTING
TIME: 25 minutes
TOTAL TIME: 53 minutes

11

Spaghetti and meat sauce are cooked in the Instant Pot to create this delicious weekday meal!

- 1 pound lean ground beef
- 1 onion diced
- 2 cloves garlic minced
- 1 cup water
- 6 ounces spaghetti uncooked
- 14 ounces diced tomatoes with juices
- 2 cups marinara sauce or pasta sauce
- ¾ cup red wine
- 1 teaspoon Italian seasoning
- ½ cup parmesan cheese grated
- 1 tablespoon parsley chopped

1. Turn a 6QT Instant Pot onto saute. Cook beef, onion and garlic until browned and no pink remains. Drain fat if there is more than 1 tablespoon or so.
2. Add water and scrape any brown bits. Break spaghetti in half and add spaghetti, tomatoes, marinara, wine, and Italian seasoning. Press the pasta so the sauce covers it.
3. Close the lid and select manual, high pressure for 8 minutes.
4. Once completed, quick release pressure and stir. Rest 5-10 minutes.
5. Stir in cheese and parsley. Serve immediately.

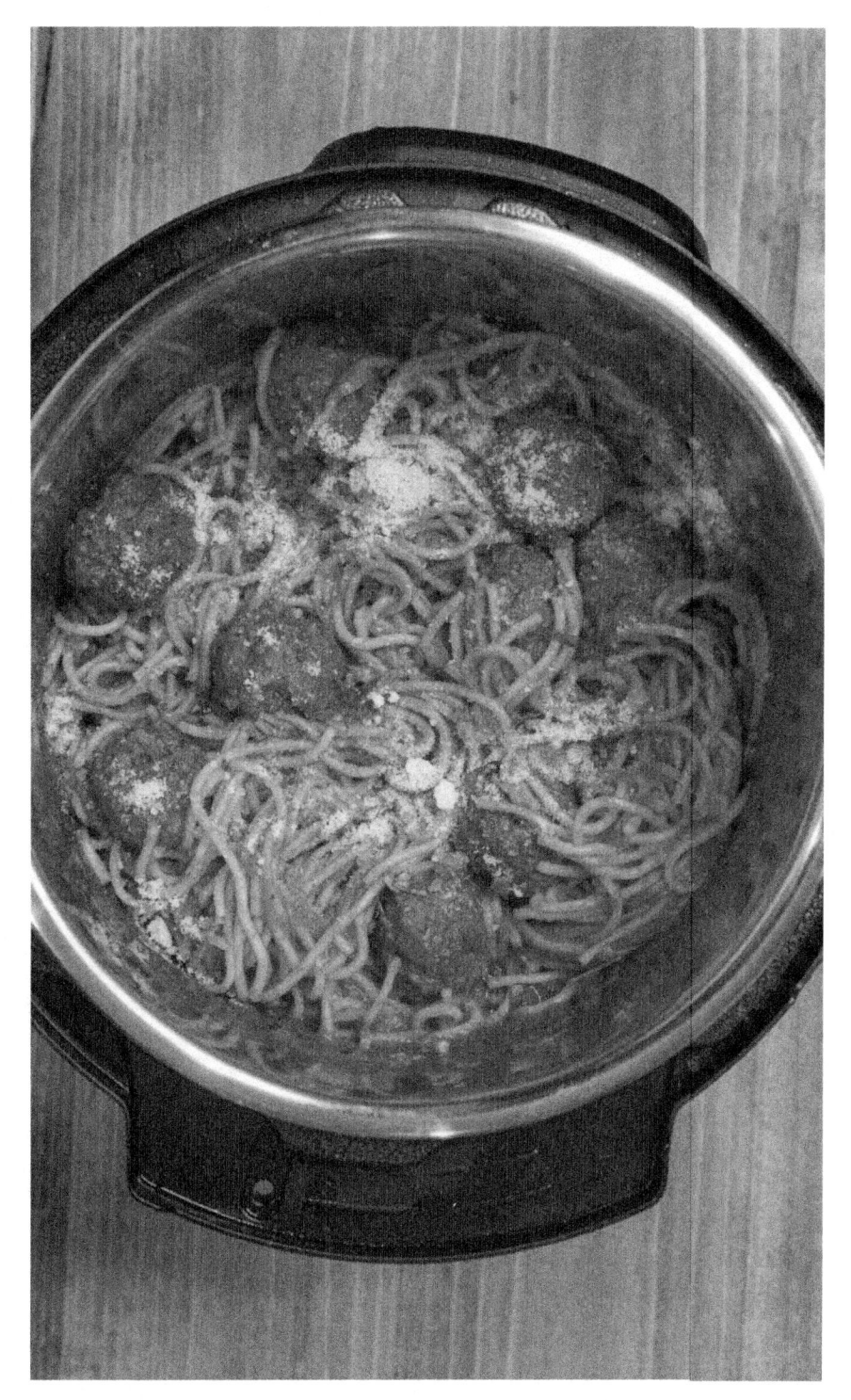

Recipe Notes

1. Deglaze the brown bits on the bottom of the pan after browning the meat, this helps avoid the dreaded burn notice!
2. Submerge Ensure the pasta is completely submerged in the sauce before cooking.
3. Size This recipe has only been tested in a 6QT Instant Pot. If your IP is a different size, consult your manual.
4. Rest Once cooked you will see liquid on the top, give it a stir an allow it to sit for at least 10 minutes uncovered. The pasta will continue to cook and the sauce will thicken.

NUTRITION FACTS

Calories: 367, Carbohydrates: 32g, Protein: 23g, Fat: 14g, Saturated Fat: 6g, Cholesterol: 57mg, Sodium: 624mg, Potassium: 753mg, Fiber: 3g, Sugar: 7g, Vitamin A: 552IU, Vitamin C: 14mg, Calcium: 161mg, Iron: 4mg

Instant Pot Pot Roast

PREP TIME: 25 minutes Serves: 6
COOK TIME: 1 hour
NATURAL RELEASE: 15 minutes
TOTAL TIME: 1 hour 40 minutes

This is a warm and tasty main dish with tender roast beef, veggies, and gravy!

- 3 pounds beef roast chuck is a great choice
- 2 tablespoons olive oil
- 1 onion diced
- ½ cup red wine
- 1 pound baby potatoes
- 3 carrots sliced into 2" pieces
- 1 stalk celery chopped into 1" pieces
- 2 sprigs fresh rosemary or 1 teaspoon dry
- 2 cloves garlic
- 2 cups beef broth
- 2 tablespoons tomato paste
- 1 bay leaf

Gravy
- ½ cup broth or water, or as needed
- 3 tablespoons cornstarch

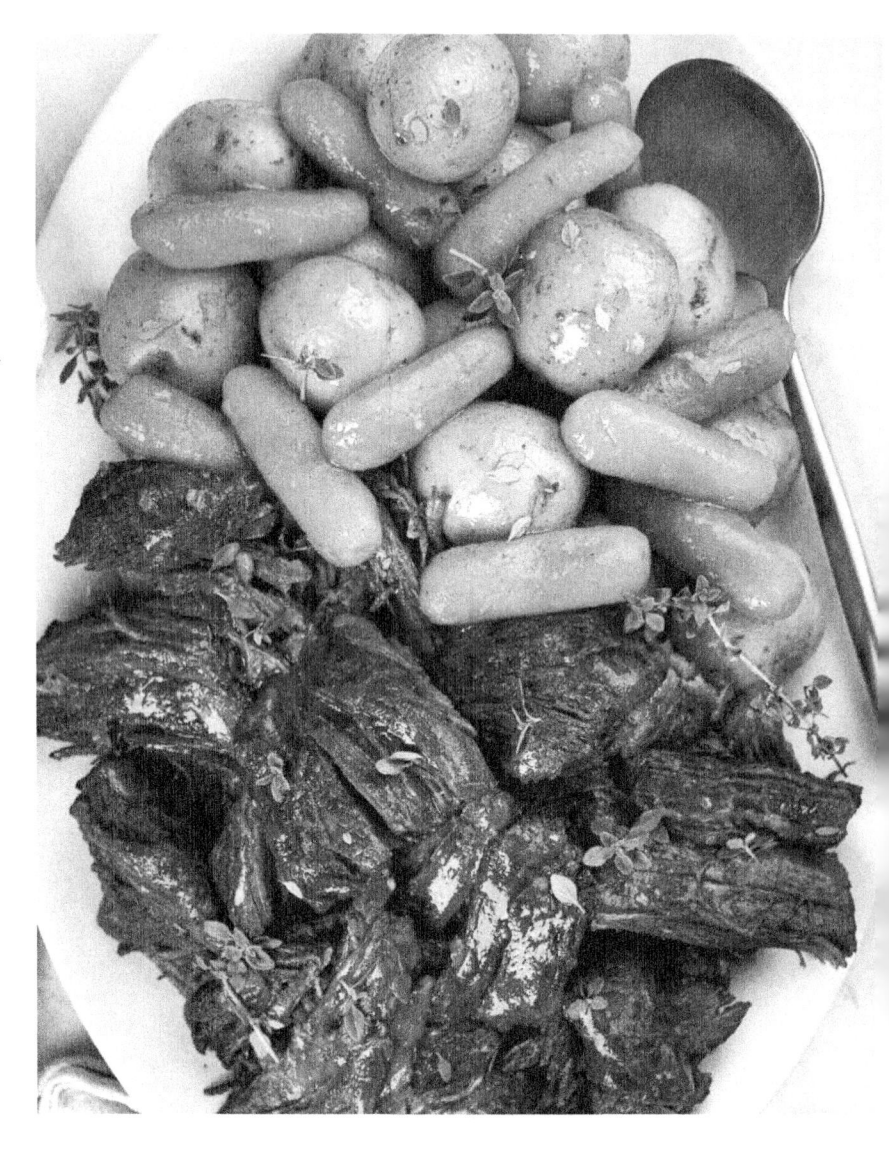

1. Cut roast into large 3 to 4" chunks. Season generously with salt & pepper.
2. Add olive oil to the Instant Pot and turn on to saute. Sear beef in batches to brown, about 4 minutes per side.
3. Remove beef and add onions to the Instant Pot (you can add a bit more oil if needed). Cook 2-3 minutes to soften.
4. Add red wine to the Instant Pot. Scrape the bottom to remove any brown bits (to avoid a burn notice).
5. Add remaining ingredients and mix well. Add browned beef and stir.
6. Cook on high pressure for 45 minutes. Natural release 15 minutes.
7. Using a slotted spoon, remove beef and vegetables and set on a plate to rest. Discard bay leaf.
8. Combine broth and cornstarch in a mason jar and shake very well until smooth. Turn the broth in the Instant Pot onto saute to bring to a boil. Whisk in cornstarch and cook until thickened and bubbly, add additional cornstarch as necessary. Season with salt and pepper.
9. Serve gravy over pot roast.

NUTRITION FACTS

Calories: 436, Carbohydrates: 24g, Protein: 53g, Fat: 13g, Saturated Fat: 3g, Cholesterol: 129mg, Sodium: 3636mg, Potassium: 1334mg, Fiber: 3g, Sugar: 4g, Vitamin A: 5207IU, Vitamin C: 122mg, Calcium: 665mg, Iron: 6mg

Instant Pot Lentil Soup

PREP TIME: 25 minutes Serves: 8
COOK TIME: 15 minutes
NATURAL RELEASE: 10 minutes
TOTAL TIME: 50 minutes

Pressure cooked with ground beef and vegetables, this is a tasty and hearty soup that just takes minutes to prepare!

- 1 pound ground beef
- 2 cloves garlic minced
- 1 onion diced
- 1 tablespoon olive oil
- 1 cup celery sliced
- 1 cup carrots sliced
- 1 large baking potato peeled and cubed
- 1 cup lentils
- 6 cups beef broth
- 28 oz diced tomatoes with juices
- 1 tablespoon Worcestershire sauce
- 1 teaspoon Italian seasoning
- salt and pepper to taste
- fresh parsley and parmesan cheese for garnish optional

1. Turn a 6QT Instant Pot onto saute. Cook beef, onion, and garlic until browned and no pink remains. Drain fat if there is more than 1 tablespoon or so. While beef is browning, prepare vegetables.
2. Add beef broth and scrape up any brown bits on the bottom of the pan. Add remaining ingredients.
3. Set instant pot to high pressure for 15 minutes. Once the instant pot has cooked for 15 minutes, allow it to naturally release for 10 minutes. Release remaining pressure.
4. Serve with parmesan cheese & parsley if desired.

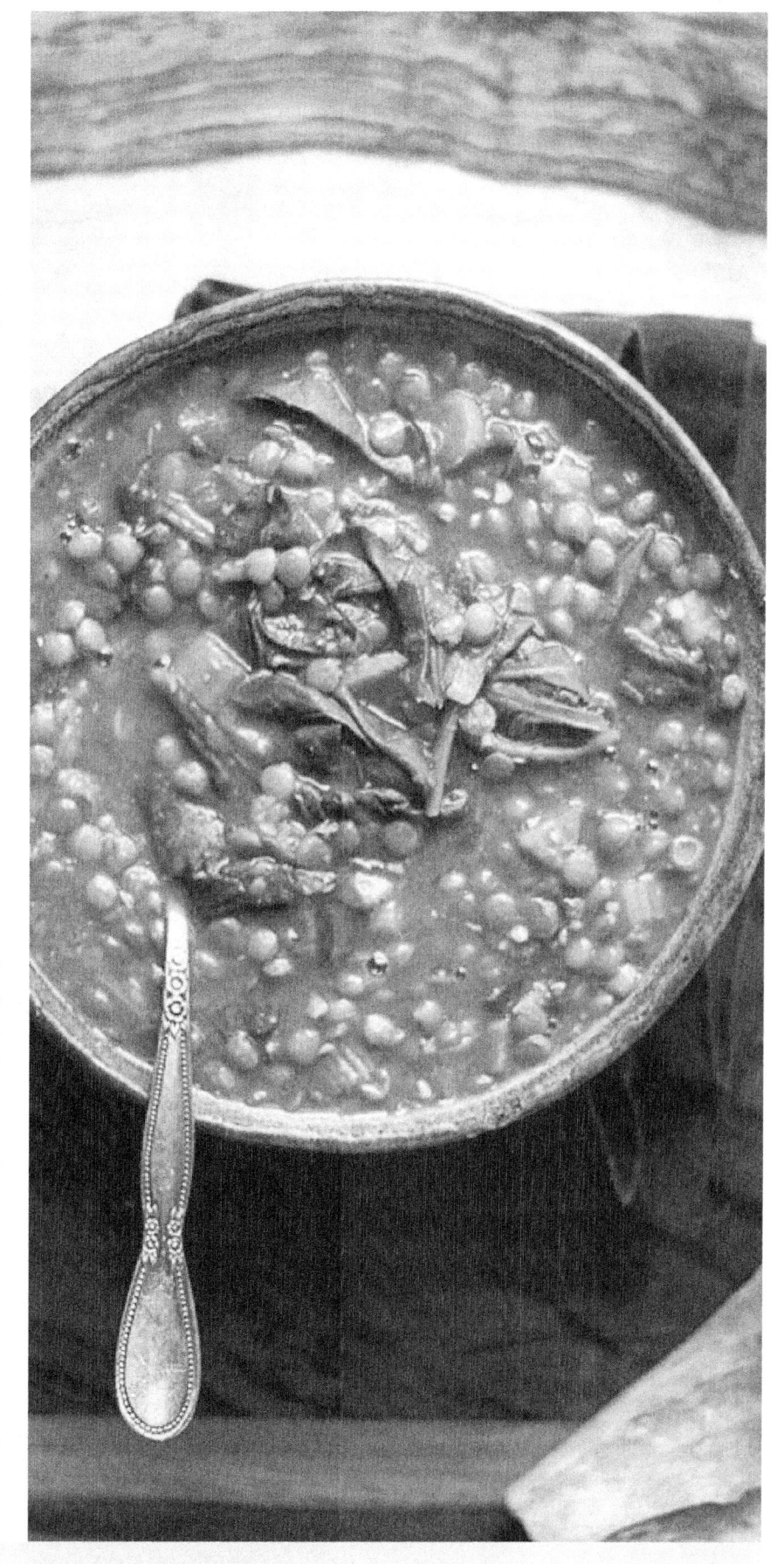

NUTRITION FACTS

Serving: 1.5cups, Calories: 245, Carbohydrates: 27g, Protein: 23g, Fat: 5g, Saturated Fat: 2g, Cholesterol: 35mg, Sodium: 555mg, Potassium: 1204mg, Fiber: 10g, Sugar: 5g, Vitamin A: 2855IU, Vitamin C: 15mg, Calcium: 74mg, Iron: 5mg

Instant Pot Mushroom Risotto

PREP TIME: 15 minutes
COOK TIME: 20 minutes
TOTAL TIME: 35 minutes
Serves: 4

9

Creamy & savory, this Instant Pot Mushroom Risotto is sure to be a hit with the whole family!

- 1 tablespoon olive oil
- 1 small onion finely chopped
- 8 ounces mushrooms sliced
- 1 cup arborio rice
- ¼ cup white wine
- 2 cups chicken broth
- 2 cloves garlic minced
- ¼ teaspoon dried thyme
- ¼ teaspoon salt
- ⅛ teaspoon black pepper
- 1 tablespoon butter
- ¼ cup Parmesan cheese shredded, divided

1. Heat olive oil in the Instant Pot using the saute setting.
2. Add onions and mushrooms. Cook 3-4 minutes or until mushrooms are tender.
3. Add the rice and cook for 2-3 minutes. Add white wine and scrape any brown bits off the bottom of the Instant Pot.
4. Stir in broth, garlic and seasonings. Place the lid on the Instant Pot and turn the valve to seal. Set to pressure cook on high for 5 minutes.
5. Once the cook time is off, let it sit without opening the lid for 10 minutes (natural release). After 10 minutes release any remaining pressure and open the lid.
6. Stir in butter and 2 tablespoons parmesan cheese.
7. Serve and garnish with remaining parmesan cheese.

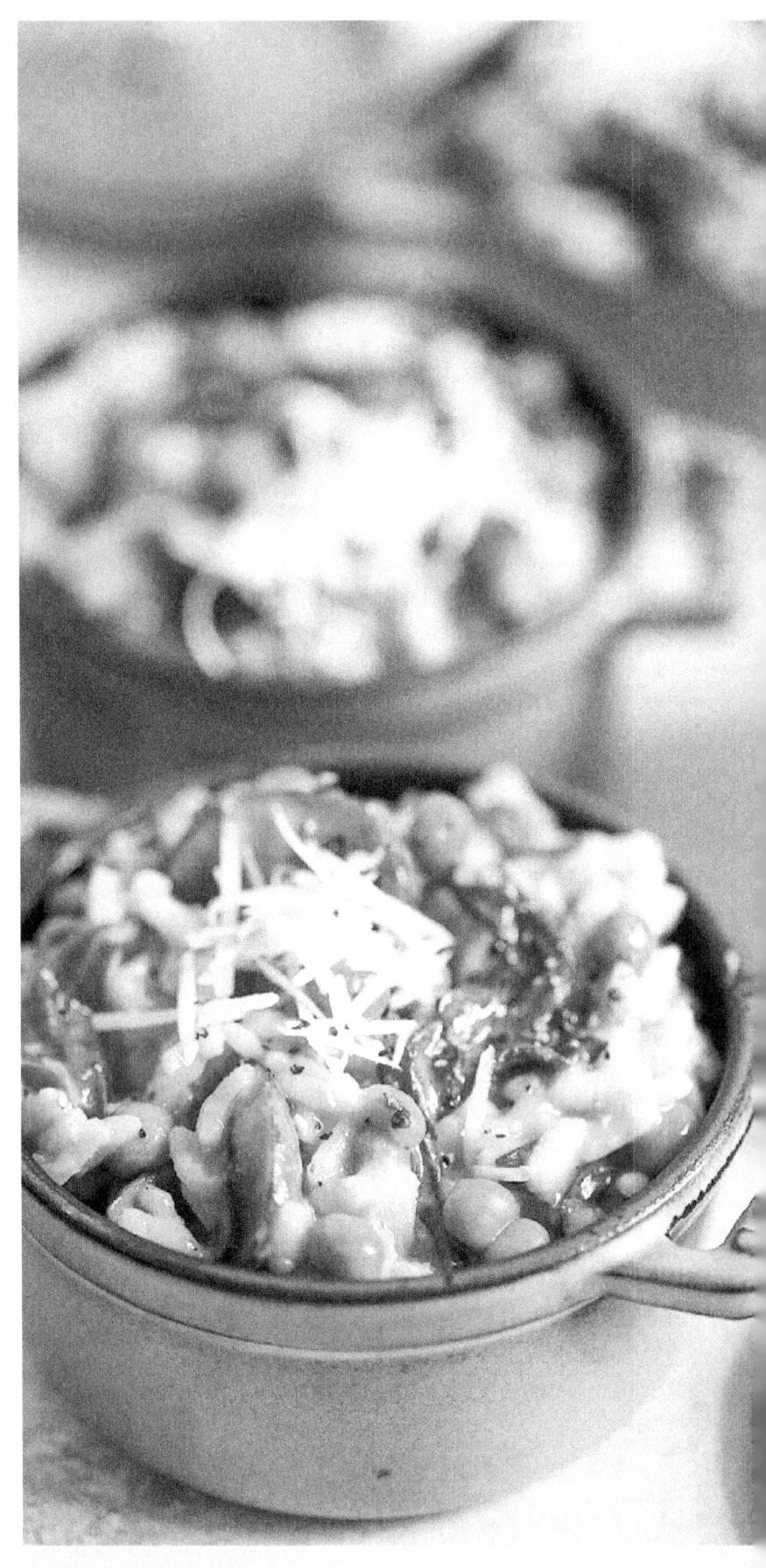

NUTRITION FACTS

Calories: 300, Carbohydrates: 45g, Protein: 8g, Fat: 9g, Saturated Fat: 3g, Cholesterol: 12mg, Sodium: 706mg, Potassium: 349mg, Fiber: 2g, Sugar: 2g, Vitamin A: 136IU, Vitamin C: 11mg, Calcium: 88mg, Iron: 3mg

Instant Pot Turkey Breast

PREP TIME: 10 minutes
COOK TIME: 27 minutes
NATURAL RELEASE: 10 minutes
TOTAL TIME: 47 minutes

Serves: 6

9

This Instant Pot Turkey Breast comes out juicy, tender, and perfectly seasoned every time!

- 1 turkey breast 3 pounds, boneless with skin
- 2 tablespoons olive oil
- ½ onion sliced
- 1 ½ cups chicken broth
- few sprigs of fresh herbs parsley, rosemary, sage, and/or thyme

For Gravy (Optional)
- 2 tablespoons each flour and butter or 2 tablespoons corn starch
- ½ teaspoon poultry seasoning optional

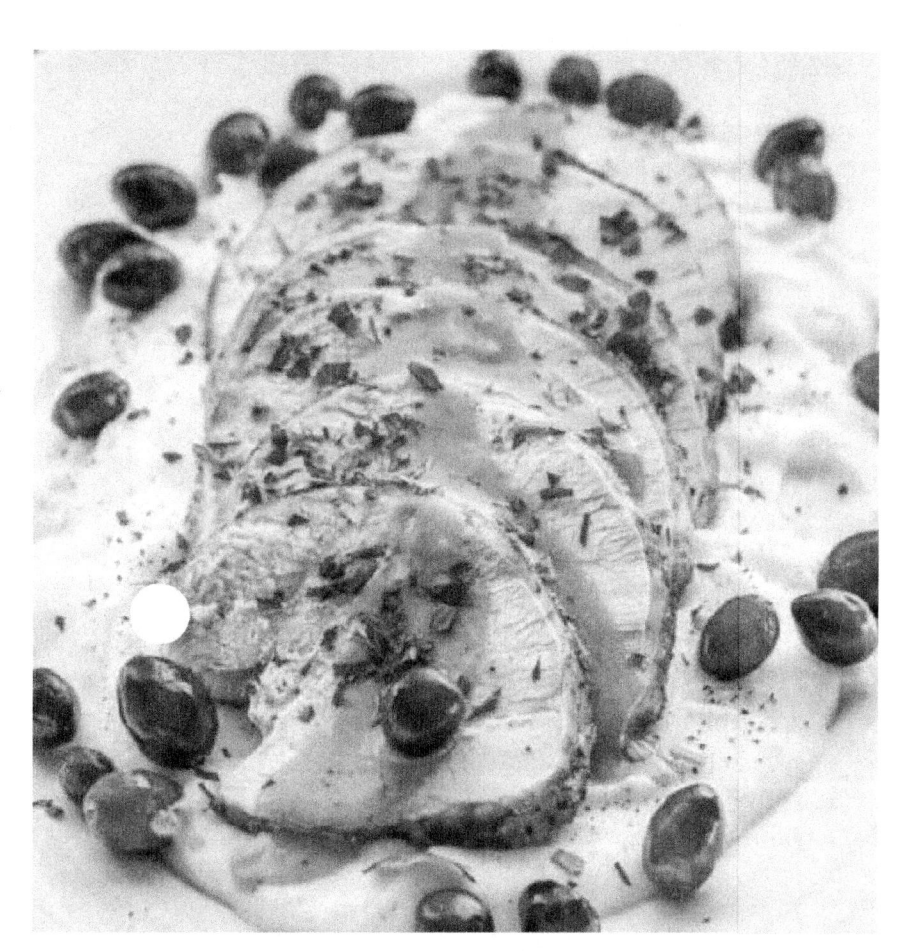

1. Season the turkey breast with salt & pepper. Turn the Instant Pot on to Saute and add oil.
2. Once the oil is hot, add the turkey breast, skin side down. Allow to cook for 5-6 minutes or until browned.
3. Remove the turkey from the Instant Pot and add broth. Scrape any brown bits off the bottom.
4. Place the onion slices and herbs in the bottom of the Instant Pot with the broth. Add the trivet.
5. Place the turkey breast, skin side up, on the trivet.
6. Set the Instant Pot to high pressure for 22 minutes. Once the cycle is completed, allow the turkey to naturally release for 10 minutes. Release any remaining pressure.
7. Use a thermometer to ensure the turkey breast has reached an internal temperature of 165°F. For a crispy skin, place the turkey under the broiler for 3-4 minutes.

To Make Gravy with Flour (cornstarch directions in the notes)

1. Remove broth and strain. Set aside.
2. Turn the Instant Pot on to saute and combine 2 tablespoons butter, 2 tablespoons flour, and poultry seasoning if using. Cook in the Instant Pot for 1 minute while stirring.
3. Add the strained broth a little bit at a time, whisking after each addition, to reach desired thickness. It will be thick at first but will thin out.
4. Season gravy with salt and pepper to taste (and stir in additional fresh herbs if desired).

NUTRITION FACTS

Calories: 190, Carbohydrates: 4g, Protein: 28g, Fat: 7g, Saturated Fat: 1g, Cholesterol: 70mg, Sodium: 484mg, Potassium: 375mg, Fiber: 1g, Sugar: 1g, Vitamin A: 26IU, Vitamin C: 5mg, Calcium: 24mg, Iron: 1mg

Instant Pot Egg Bites

PREP TIME: 5 minutes
COOK TIME: 8 minutes
TOTAL TIME: 13 minutes
Serves: 7

2

These Instant Pot Egg Bites are an easy and healthy breakfast made in the pressure cooker!

- 5 eggs
- ¼ cup milk
- ¼ teaspoon salt
- 1 pinch black pepper
- ¼ cup ham chopped
- ¼ cup cheddar cheese shredded
- 1 tablespoon green onions sliced
- 1 cup water

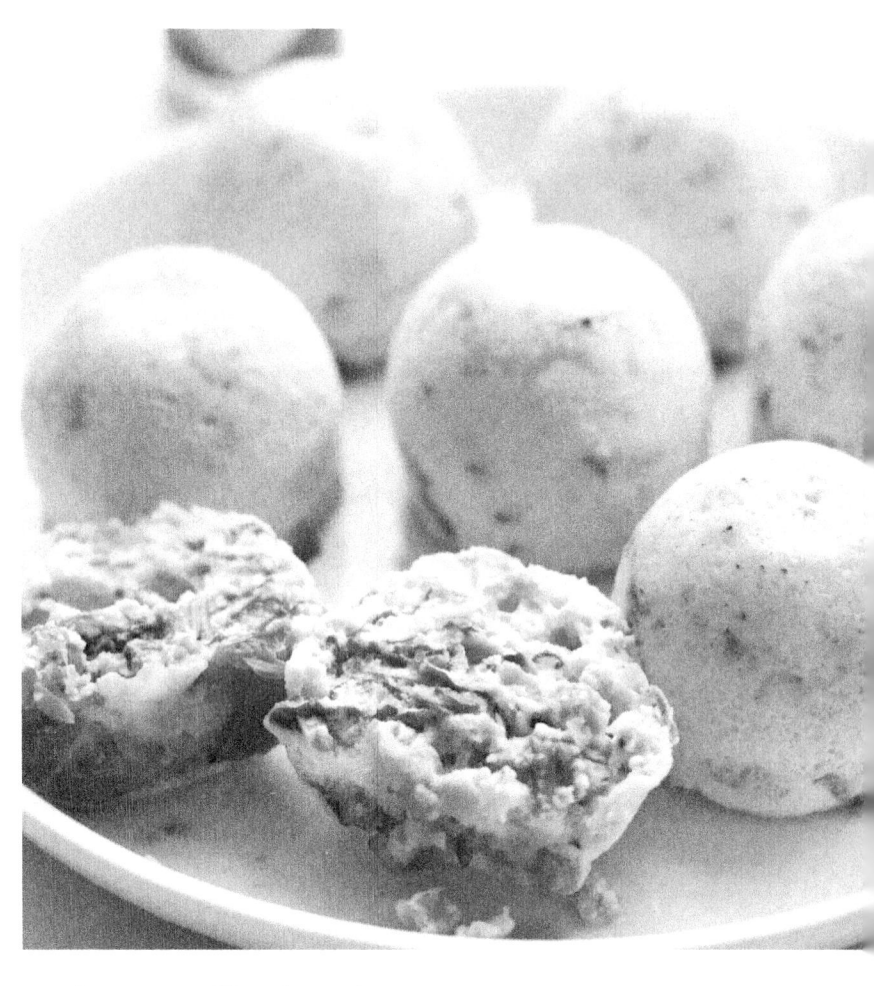

1. In a medium liquid measuring cup, whisk together eggs, milk, salt, and pepper.
2. Grease a silicone 7 egg bite mold with non stick spray and divide egg mixture between cups.
3. Divide ham, cheese, and green onion between cups - no need to stir! They will sink down.
4. Place cover on mold or wrap tightly with tin foil. Place mold on trivet.
5. Pour water (1.5 cups for an 8 quart) into the Instant Pot liner and lower the trivet with the mold into the Instant Pot.
6. Put the lid on, turn the valve to sealing, and select Manual or Pressure Cook, high pressure for 8 minutes. It will take 5-10 minutes to come to pressure and begin counting down.
7. Once the cook time is up, turn the Instant Pot off and let the pressure release naturally for 10 minutes before opening the valve to release remaining pressure.
8. Pull trivet and mold out of Instant Pot, unwrap, and gently pop egg bites out of mold onto a plate. They will be hot!
9. As they cool they may deflate slightly, but they will still be delicious.

Recipe Notes
1. Instant Pot Egg Bites will keep in the fridge in an airtight container for up to 7 days.
2. To reheat, microwave for 30 second intervals until heated through.
3. They can also be frozen and reheated in the microwave for 1-2 minutes or until heated through.

NUTRITION FACTS

Calories: 77, Carbohydrates: 1g, Protein: 6g, Fat: 5g, Saturated Fat: 2g, Cholesterol: 125mg, Sodium: 218mg, Potassium: 70mg, Sugar: 1g, Vitamin A: 235IU, Vitamin C: 1mg, Calcium: 57mg, Iron: 1mg

Instant Pot Risotto

PREP TIME: 5 minutes
COOK TIME: 5 minutes
PRESSURE RELEASE: 10 minutes
TOTAL TIME: 20 minutes

Serves: 4

9

This Instant Pot Risotto is perfect for a weekday side dish! Tender and creamy, incredibly flavorful risotto in 20 minutes!

- 2 tablespoons butter
- ½ onion finely chopped
- 1 cup arborio rice
- 1 teaspoon garlic
- ¼ teaspoon dried thyme
- ¼ teaspoon salt
- ⅛ teaspoon black pepper
- 2 cups low sodium chicken broth
- 2 tablespoons freshly grated Parmesan cheese
- Optional: crispy bacon and peas for topping

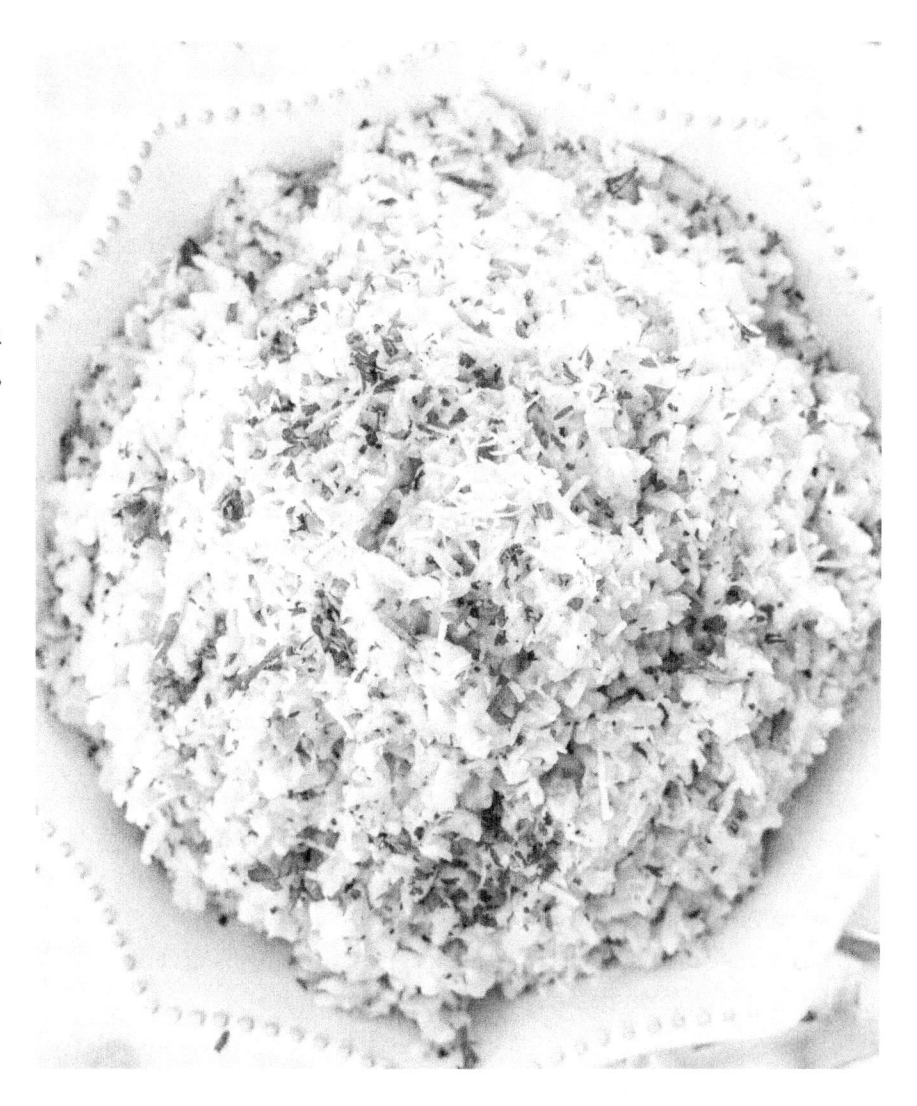

1. Turn the Instant Pot to saute and add the butter and onions.
2. Cook and stir until onions are translucent.
3. Add the rice, garlic, thyme, salt, and pepper and cook for 2-3 minutes, stirring often, until the edges of the rice are just translucent.
4. Add the chicken broth to pot and scrape the bottom well to remove any bits that may be stuck on.
5. Turn the Instant Pot off, and with the vent in the venting position, put the lid on. Turn the valve to sealing, select Manual or Pressure Cook for 5 minutes. The Instant Pot will take about 5 minutes to build pressure and begin counting down.
6. When the cook time is over, turn the Instant Pot off and let the pressure release naturally for at least 10 minutes. Open the vent, then remove the lid.
7. Stir in Parmesan cheese and any toppings as desired.

NUTRITION FACTS

Calories: 266, Carbohydrates: 43g, Protein: 7g, Fat: 7g, Saturated Fat: 4g, Cholesterol: 17mg, Sodium: 270mg, Potassium: 160mg, Fiber: 2g, Sugar: 1g, Vitamin A: 197IU, Vitamin C: 1mg, Calcium: 36mg, Iron: 2mg

Instant Pot Cheesecake

PREP TIME: 15 minutes **Serves:** 12
COOK TIME: 34 minutes
REFRIGERATION TIME: 8 hours
TOTAL TIME 8 hours : 49 minutes

16

This Instant Pot Cheesecake is a creamy dessert that pairs perfectly with summer fruit!

- 1 ½ cups graham cracker crumbs
- ¼ cup melted butter
- 16 ounces cream cheese room temperature
- 3/4 cup granulated sugar
- 1/2 cup sour cream or Greek yogurt (plain)
- 2 large eggs room temperature
- 1 teaspoon vanilla
- 1 ½ cups water for Instant Pot

1. Preheat oven to 350°F.
2. In a medium bowl, stir together graham crumbs and butter. Press into the bottom and about 1" up the sides of a 7" springform pan or push pan.
3. Bake crust for 10 minutes, or until dry. Set aside to cool slightly.
4. In a large bowl, beat cream cheese with an electric mixer on medium speed until smooth.
5. Add sugar and beat on low speed until smooth. Using low speed helps to prevent adding unnecessary air bubbles to the batter.
6. Add sour cream and beat on low speed just until smooth.
7. Add eggs and vanilla and beat on low speed until smooth.
8. Pour into prepared crust. Tap gently on the counter to bring air bubbles to the top and pop with a knife.
9. Tear off a long piece of foil and fold it lengthwise to create a long narrow sling.
10. Pour the water into the Instant Pot, then place the trivet in the pot. Put the sling on top of the trivet, bending it to lay flat on the bottom and stick up the sides, as shown in the image above.
11. Place pan on top of the sling, and fold the ends of the sling over top the pan.
12. Put the lid on, turn the valve to sealing, and select Pressure Cook for 32 minutes. It will take about 10 minutes to build pressure.
13. When the cook time is over, turn the Instant Pot off and allow the pressure to release naturally before opening the valve and removing the lid.
14. Remove the pan from the Instant Pot using the sling. Set on a wire rack to cool to room temperature before refrigerating for 8 hours or overnight.
15. Slice and serve.

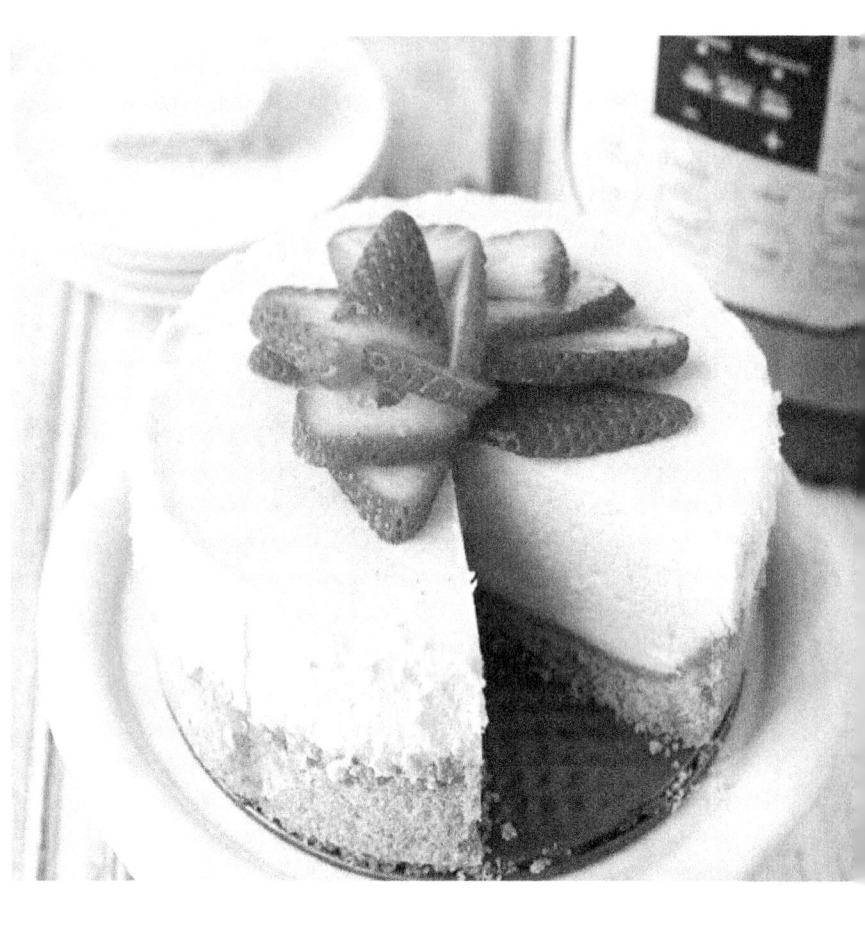

NUTRITION FACTS

Calories: 344, Carbohydrates: 27g, Protein: 5g, Fat: 25g, Saturated Fat: 14g, Cholesterol: 108mg, Sodium: 265mg, Potassium: 126mg, Fiber: 1g, Sugar: 21g, Vitamin A: 864IU, Vitamin C: 1mg, Calcium: 85mg, Iron: 1mg

Instant Pot Ribs

PREP TIME: 15 minutes **Serves:** 4
COOK TIME: 45 minutes
TOTAL TIME: 1 hour

Tender fall off the bone baby back ribs are made easy in the Instant Pot! Add your favorite barbecue sauce (or olive oil/salt/pepper) for a finger licking good meal!

- 1 rack baby back ribs about 1 ½- 2 pounds
- 1 cup broth or water
- ½ teaspoon liquid smoke optional
- 4 cloves garlic sliced
- 1 onion sliced
- 6 tablespoons dry rub
- barbecue sauce optional

Dry Rub
- 2 tablespoons paprika
- 2 tablespoons brown sugar
- 2 teaspoons garlic powder
- 2 teaspoons onion powder
- 1 teaspoon black pepper
- 2 teaspoons lemon pepper
- 1 teaspoon smoked paprika
- 2 teaspoons oregano

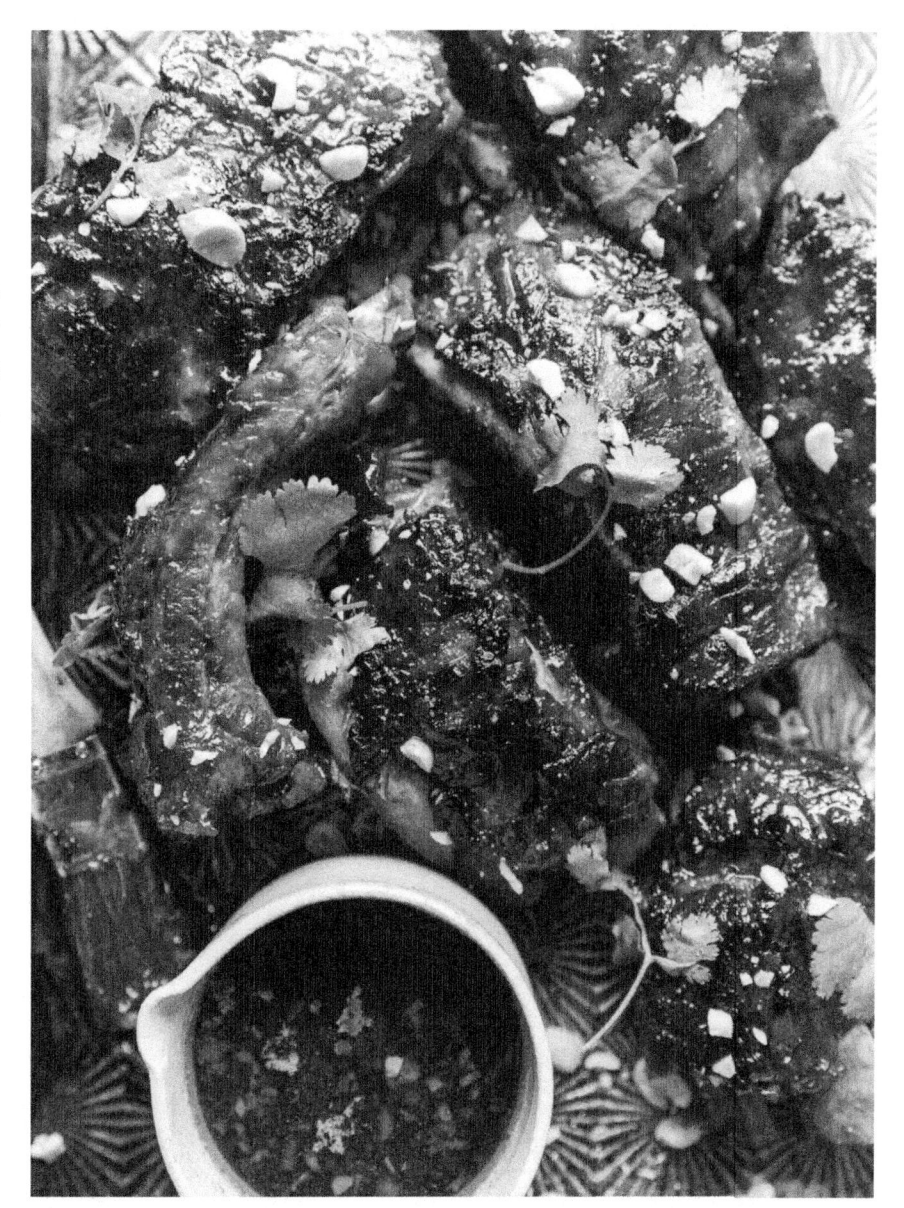

1. Rinse ribs and pat dry. Remove the thin membrane from the back of the ribs.
2. Cut slab into 2-3 pieces (enough so they fit into the Instant Pot) and coat with dry rub massaging it into the meat.
3. Place trivet (or rack) in the bottom of your Instant Pot. Add broth or water and liquid smoke if using.
4. Set ribs upright on the trivet (so they are not stacked on top of one another). Sprinkle with onion and garlic.
5. Close lid and select manual pressure and set the timer for 23 minutes (25 minutes if they're extra meaty). Once done, allow the instant pot to natural release for 5 minutes.
6. Open valve to release remaining pressure.
7. Brush with barbecue sauce (or olive oil/salt/pepper for dry ribs) and broil or grill until slightly charred.

NUTRITION FACTS

Calories: 244, Carbohydrates: 19g, Protein: 15g, Fat: 12g, Saturated Fat: 4g, Cholesterol: 48mg, Sodium: 307mg, Potassium: 413mg, Fiber: 3g, Sugar: 8g, Vitamin A: 2285IU, Vitamin C: 4mg, Calcium: 131mg, Iron: 4.2mg

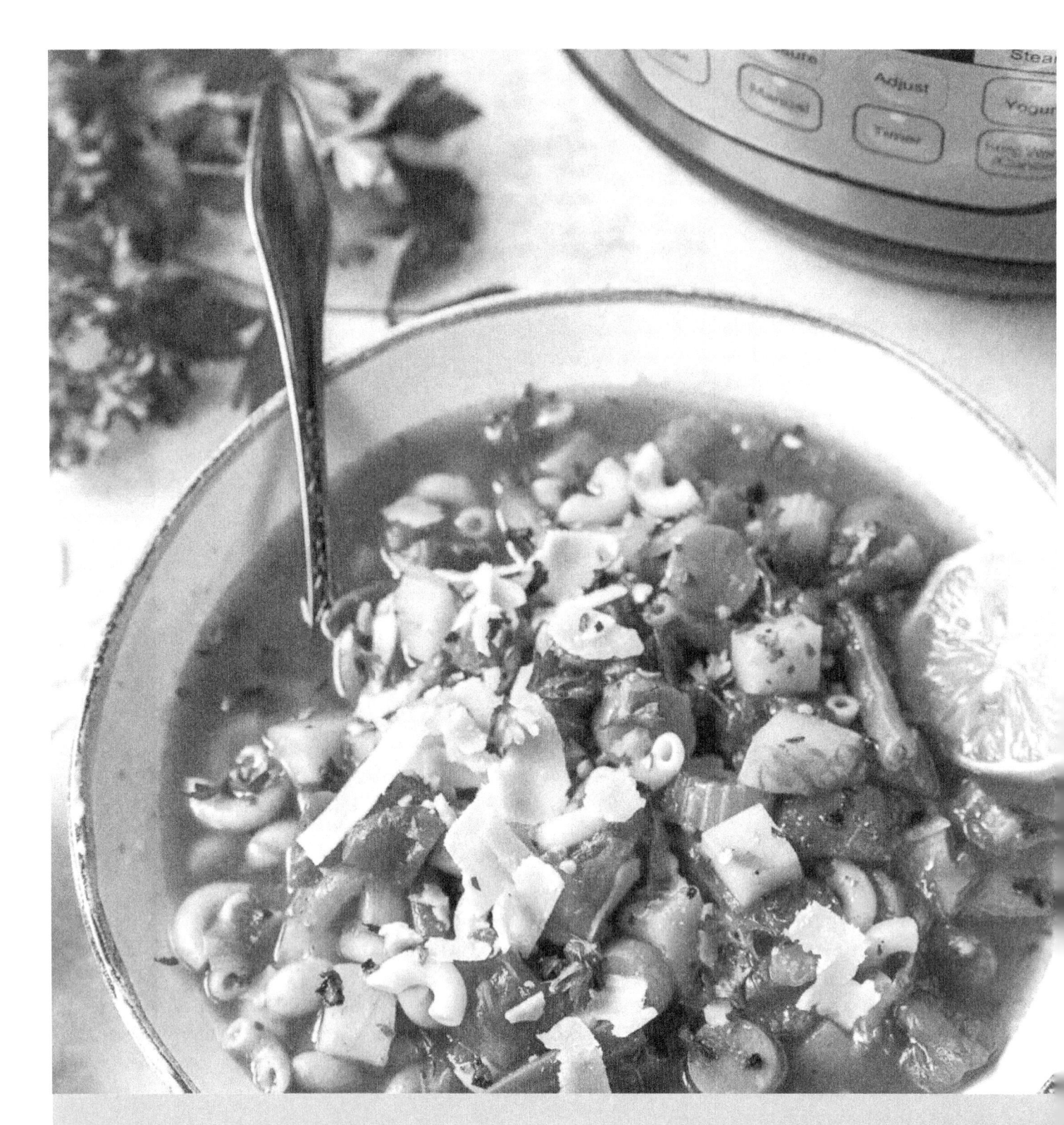

Chapter 9:
Dip & Dressing

Baked Taco Ground Beef Dip

PREP TIME: 20 minutes   Serves: 6
COOK TIME: 45 minutes
TOTAL TIME: 1 hour 5 minutes

`20`

Make this appetizer for a party or potluck & serve warm out of the oven with tortilla chips!

- 1 pound ground beef or ground turkey or ground chicken
- 1 package taco seasoning
- 8 ounces cream cheese softened
- ¼ cup sour cream
- 2 cups cheddar cheese shredded, divided
- 1 cup Monterey jack cheese shredded, divided
- 2 ounces green chilis chopped
- 1 cup salsa

Optional Toppings
- lettuce
- tomatoes
- olives
- cilantro
- jalapenos
- green onions

1. Preheat oven to 375°F.
2. Brown beef in a large pan over medium heat, drain fat and return to the pan.
3. Stir in taco seasoning and water according to package directions.
4. While beef is cooking mix cream cheese, sour cream, ½ of the cheese, and chilis in a large bowl. Mix until fully combined and spread into the bottom of a baking dish.
5. Layer the meat mixture on top, then layer the salsa and finish with the remaining cheese
6. Bake 25 minutes or until bubbly and browned. Top with desired toppings and serve warm with chips.

Recipe Notes

1. Remember to soften the cream cheese. This will make it easier to mix with the other ingredients. Let it soften on the counter, or do it in the microwave on a lower power for about 45 seconds.
2. Use a hand mixer to combine the cream cheese mixture, this makes the dip easier to scoop.
3. Make this up to 2 days ahead and bake just before the guests arrive.
4. Top with your favorite toppings. (Sour cream, tomatoes, green onions, shredded lettuce, black olives, cilantro etc).

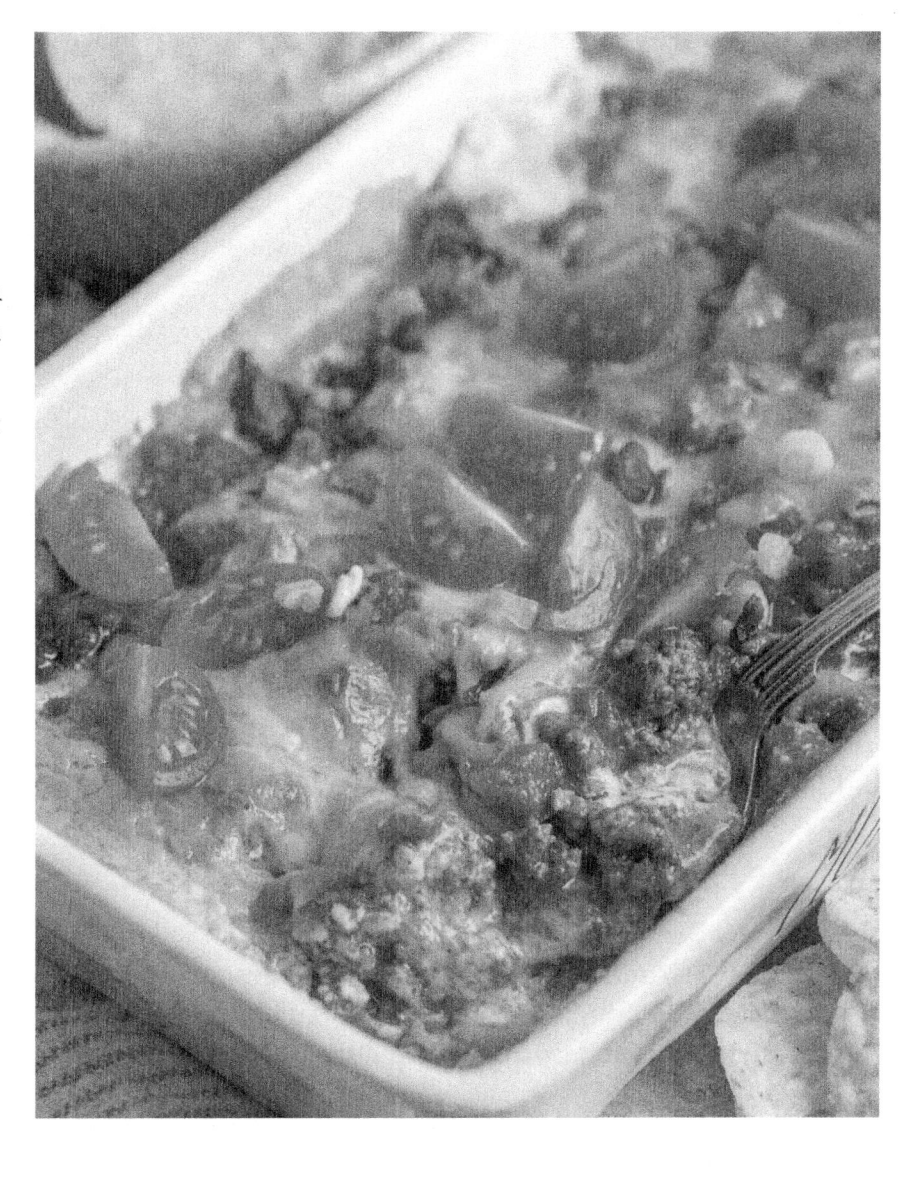

NUTRITION FACTS

Calories: 499, Carbohydrates: 9g, Protein: 33g, Fat: 37g, Saturated Fat: 22g, Polyunsaturated Fat: 1g, Monounsaturated Fat: 11g, Trans Fat: 1g, Cholesterol: 150mg, Sodium: 1321mg, Potassium: 503mg, Fiber: 2g, Sugar: 5g, Vitamin A: 1845IU, Vitamin C: 5mg, Calcium: 479mg, Iron: 3mg

Easy Buffalo Chicken Dip (with canned chicken)

PREP TIME: 15 minutes
COOK TIME: 20 minutes
TOTAL TIME: 35 minutes

Serves: 8

11

A rich, creamy, & cheesy dip with buffalo wing-inspired flavors, baked to bubbly perfection!

- 8 ounces cream cheese softened
- ½ cup sour cream
- 1 packet ranch mix
- 12 oz canned cooked chicken, drained or 2 cups shredded chicken
- 2 cups cheddar cheese or Monterey jack, shredded, divided
- ½ cup buffalo sauce

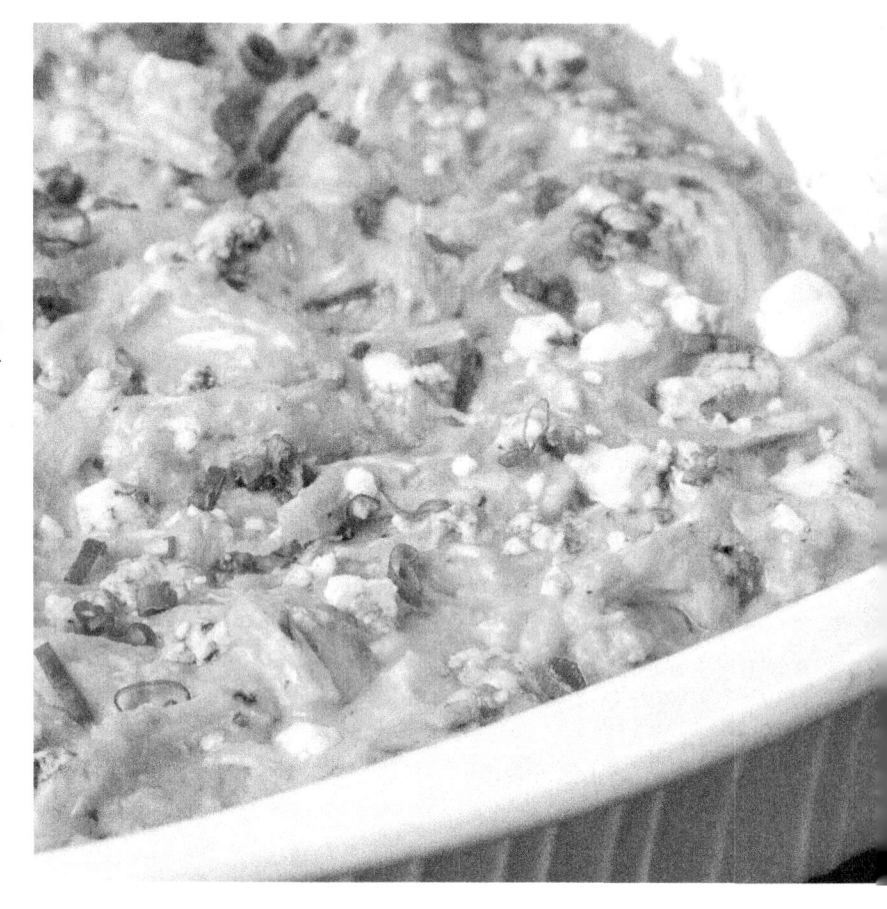

1. Preheat oven to 350°F.
2. Combine cream cheese, sour cream, ranch mix and 1 cup of the cheese with a mixer.
3. Spread into the bottom of a 1 ½ qt baking dish.
4. Top with chicken, buffalo sauce, and remaining cheese.
5. Bake 20 minutes or until hot and bubbly.

Recipe Notes
1. Optional toppings and add-ins: chopped celery, green onions, parsley, garlic powder, blue cheese crumbles
2. Make-Ahead: This dip can easily be made 48 hours ahead of time and refrigerated for perfect party planning.
3. Use a Hand Mixer: Using a hand mixer for the cream cheese base makes is soft and scoopable!
4. Feed a Crowd: This recipe can easily be doubled (or tripled) to feed a crowd. Cook time may need to be increased.
5. Toppings: I've kept this simple but you can add in your own favorite toppings. Blue cheese, green onions, bacon bits, or crispy fried onions are all great on this buffalo dip!
6. Tailgating: Spread this into a disposable pan and cook over indirect heat on the grill. You can also make buffalo chicken dip in the crockpot.
7. Store leftover dip in the fridge in an airtight container for up to 3 days.
8. Reheat in the oven or in the microwave until heated through.

NUTRITION FACTS

Calories: 248, Carbohydrates: 4g, Protein: 9g, Fat: 22g, Saturated Fat: 13g, Cholesterol: 68mg, Sodium: 1004mg, Potassium: 87mg, Sugar: 1g, Vitamin A: 753IU, Vitamin C: 1mg, Calcium: 247mg, Iron: 1mg

Easy Cheesy Pizza Dip

PREP TIME: 15 minutes
COOK TIME: 30 minutes
TOTAL TIME: 45 minutes

Serves: 8

`10`

Easy Cheesy Pizza Dip is so delicious & creamy! Serve hot from the oven with tortilla chips or bread to impress a crowd.

- 8 ounces cream cheese softened
- 2 cups mozzarella cheese shredded, divided
- ½ cup cheddar cheese shredded
- ½ teaspoon dried oregano
- ¼ teaspoon dried basil
- 1 cup pizza sauce
- ¼ cup fresh parmesan cheese shredded
- pepperoni slices to taste, approx ¼ cup
- tortilla chips or 1 loaf of sourdough bread cut into cubes for serving

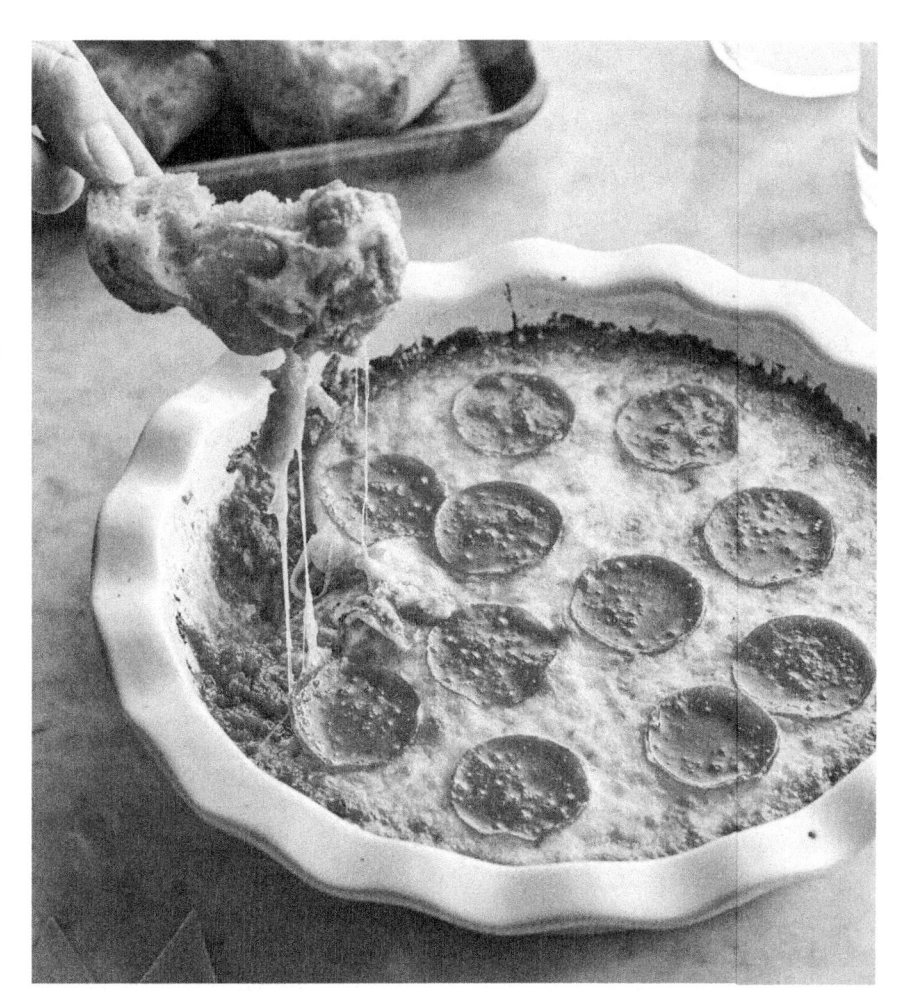

1. Preheat oven to 350°F.
2. Mix cream cheese, ¾ cup mozzarella cheese, cheddar cheese, oregano, & basil, and salt to taste.
3. Spread into a pie pan or 2qt casserole dish. Top the cream cheese mixture with pizza sauce.
4. Sprinkle remaining cheeses followed by pepperoni.
5. Bake 25 minutes or until bubbly and cheese is browned.
6. Cool 5 minutes before serving. Serve with tortilla chips or cubed bread.

Recipe Notes

1. Soften the cream cheese before mixing.
2. Use a hand mixer to make a fluffy dip that's easier to scoop.
3. I like to put the pepperoni on top of the cheese so it gets crispy.
4. To save time, buy pre-shredded cheese, it works well in this dip.
5. Allow the dip to cool at least 5 minutes before serving.
6. If adding fresh basil, add it after baking.

NUTRITION FACTS

Calories: 229, Carbohydrates: 4g, Protein: 11g, Fat: 19g, Saturated Fat: 11g, Polyunsaturated Fat: 1g, Monounsaturated Fat: 5g, Cholesterol: 63mg, Sodium: 521mg, Potassium: 174mg, Fiber: 1g, Sugar: 3g, Vitamin A: 800IU, Vitamin C: 2mg, Calcium: 264mg, Iron: 1mg

Easy Cheese Dip

PREP TIME: 5 minutes **Serves:** 8
COOK TIME: 0 minutes
CHILL (IF TIME PERMITS): 1 hour
TOTAL TIME: 5 minutes

10

Creamy and rich, with a tangy mustard bite, a 5-minute dip is perfect with your favorite crunchy snacks.

- 8 ounces cream cheese softened
- ½ cup sour cream
- ½ cup mayonnaise
- 2 cups sharp cheddar cheese shredded
- 1 teaspoon dijon mustard
- ¼ teaspoon garlic powder
- ⅛ teaspoon cayenne pepper optional

1. Combine cream cheese, sour cream and mayonnaise in a bowl with a hand mixer until fluffy.
2. Add remaining ingredients and combine until smooth.
3. For best flavor, refrigerate 1 hour if time allows.

Recipe Notes
1. Optional Add-Ins include jalapenos, pimentos, chopped artichokes, bacon bits.
2. This dip can be mixed in a food processor if desired. Pulse just until combined. If you don't have a food processor or hand mixer, mix well with a spoon.
3. This dip will last up to a week in the fridge (as long as your dairy used is fresh). Leftovers make a great filling for celery sticks or can be melted and tossed with pasta.

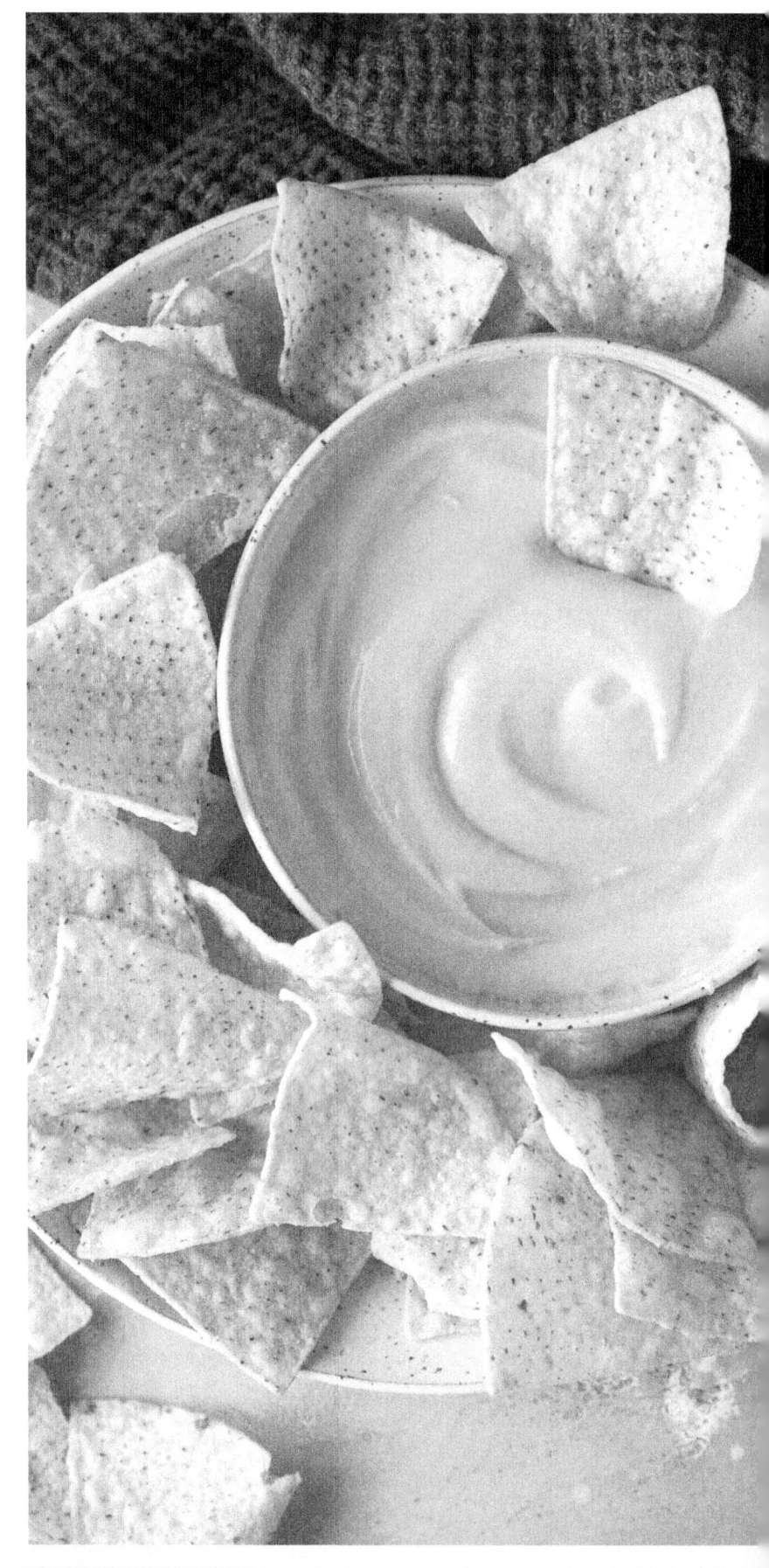

NUTRITION FACTS

Calories: 223, Carbohydrates: 1g, Protein: 6g, Fat: 22g, Saturated Fat: 10g, Cholesterol: 49mg, Sodium: 249mg, Potassium: 58mg, Sugar: 1g, Vitamin A: 517IU, Vitamin C: 1mg, Calcium: 165mg, Iron: 1mg

Buffalo Ranch Chicken Dip

PREP TIME: 15 minutes
COOK TIME: 30 minutes
TOTAL TIME: 45 minutes

Serves: 12

9

Buffalo Ranch Chicken Dip is a creamy, cheesy & spicy dip loaded with shredded chicken and lots of cheese!

- 8 ounces cream cheese softened
- ½ cup sour cream
- ½ cup ranch dressing
- 2 green onions thinly sliced
- 2 cups shredded chicken cooked
- 1 cup buffalo sauce divided
- 1 cup pepper jack cheese shredded
- 1 cup cheddar cheese shredded

1. Preheat oven to 375°F.
2. Combine cream cheese, sour cream, ranch dressing, ½ cup of the buffalo sauce, and green onions with a mixer on medium speed. Spread in a a pie plate or small casserole dish (2qt).
3. Place chicken over the cream cheese mixture and drizzle with the remaining ½ cup buffalo sauce.
4. Top with cheeses and bake 20-25 minutes or until hot & bubbly. Let cool 5 minutes before serving.

Recipe Notes
1. Ranch dressing can be substituted with additional sour cream and ranch dressing mix.
2. A hand mixer makes a fluffier dip that is easier to scoop but this can be mixed with a spoon if preferred.
3. Serve with crostini, tortilla chips, soft pretzels, or celery sticks for dipping.

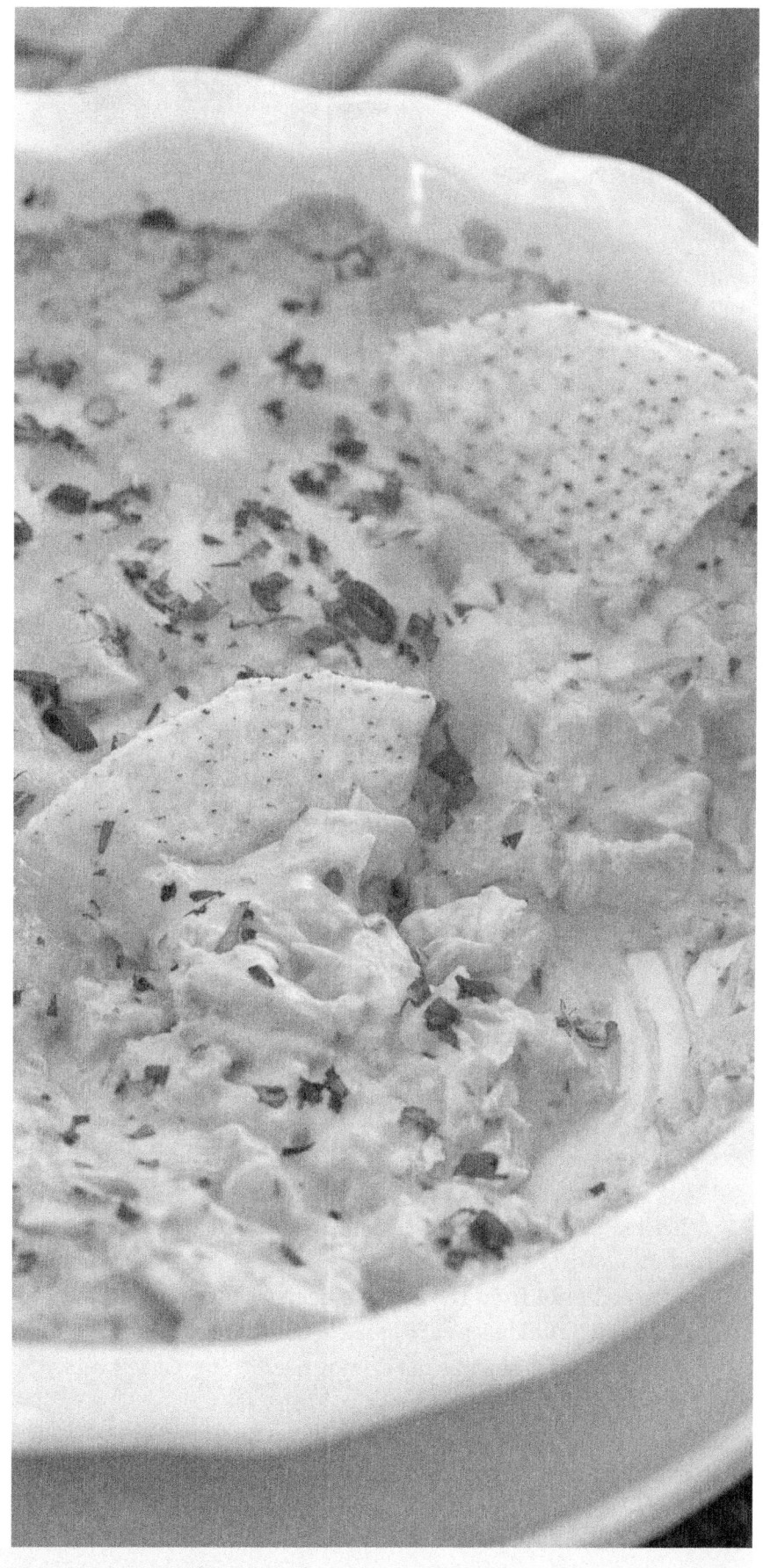

NUTRITION FACTS

Calories: 239, Carbohydrates: 1g, Protein: 11g, Fat: 21g, Saturated Fat: 9g, Cholesterol: 65mg, Sodium: 965mg, Potassium: 117mg, Sugar: 1g, Vitamin A: 490IU, Vitamin C: 0.4mg, Calcium: 173mg, Iron: 0.4mg

Quick & Easy Chocolate Hummus

PREP TIME: 10 minutes
COOK TIME: 10 minutes
TOTAL TIME: 20 minutes
Serves: 16

1

This Chocolate Hummus is a hearty & healthy dessert dip, perfect for dipping berries, salty snacks, or cookies!

- 15 ounces canned garbanzo beans (chickpeas) unsalted, juices reserved
- ⅓ cup Cacao Bliss
- 3 tablespoons tahini or peanut butter
- ⅓ tablespoon brown sugar
- 1 teaspoon vanilla
- ¼ teaspoon salt

1. Drain the garbanzo beans reserving the liquid. Rinse the beans well and place on a paper towel. Rub the beans with the paper towel to remove some of the skins.
2. Add all ingredients to a blender or food processor except reserved juices.
3. Pulse a few times to get the blending started. Add in reserved juice (3-4 tablespoons) a bit at a time until you reach desired consistency.
4. Serve with berries, cookies or pretzels.

Recipe Notes

1. Makes 2 cups, serving size 2 tablespoons.
2. This recipe uses drained garbanzo beans. If using dried garbanzo beans, cook, drain, and cool completely before using.
3. Save the liquid from the can of chickpeas (aka aquafaba) to thin out the hummus if needed. Then, freeze the rest of the liquid in ice cube trays to use in future recipes like thickening soups and sauces.
4. Chick peas/garbanzo beans do not need to be peeled but you can rub some of the skins off for a smoother texture.
5. Tahini can be replaced with another nut butter of your choice.
6. Leftover hummus can be kept in an airtight container in the fridge for up to 4 days. Mix well before serving again.

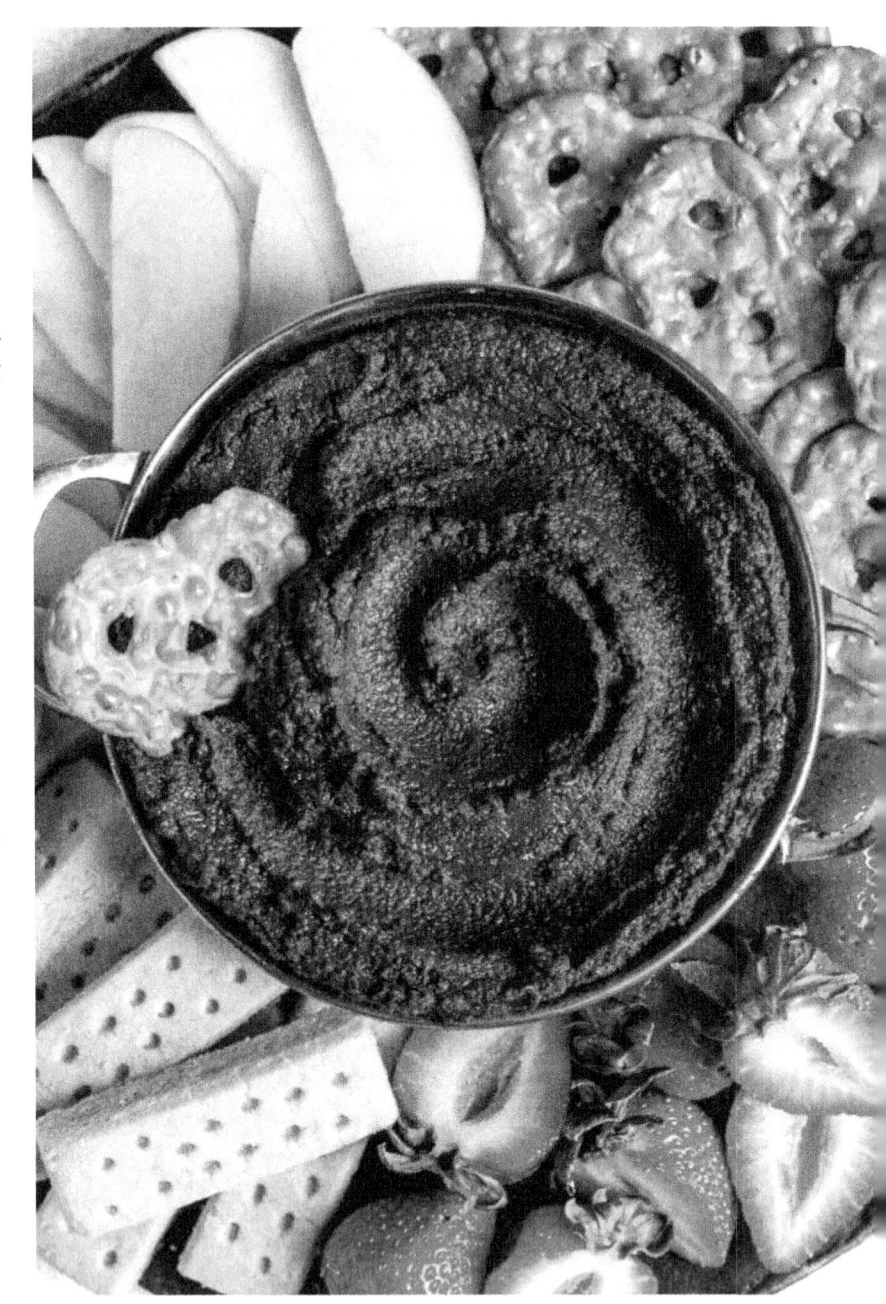

NUTRITION FACTS

Serving: 2tablespoons, Calories: 49, Carbohydrates: 5g, Protein: 3g, Fat: 2g, Saturated Fat: 1g, Polyunsaturated Fat: 1g, Monounsaturated Fat: 1g, Cholesterol: 3mg, Sodium: 121mg, Potassium: 69mg, Fiber: 2g, Sugar: 1g, Vitamin A: 6IU, Vitamin C: 1mg, Calcium: 29mg, Iron: 1mg

Fluffy Pumpkin Dip

PREP TIME: 5 minutes Serves: 8
COOK TIME: 5 minutes
CHILL TIME: 30 minutes
TOTAL TIME: 40 minutes

14

Pumpkin Pie Dip delivers fall flavors in a fluffy no-bake dip! Pumpkin & warm spices combine with a rich creamy base to make the perfect dip for apples, bananas, and more!

- 12 ounces cream cheese *
- 2 cups powdered sugar
- 1 cup canned pumpkin puree
- 1 teaspoon ground ginger
- 1 teaspoon pumpkin pie spice or cinnamon
- 2 cups whipped topping

1. Beat cream cheese and powdered sugar with a hand mixer on medium until light and fluffy. Stir in pumpkin and spices.
2. Gently fold in whipped topping. Refrigerate at least 30 minutes before serving.
3. Serve with sliced apples or graham crackers.

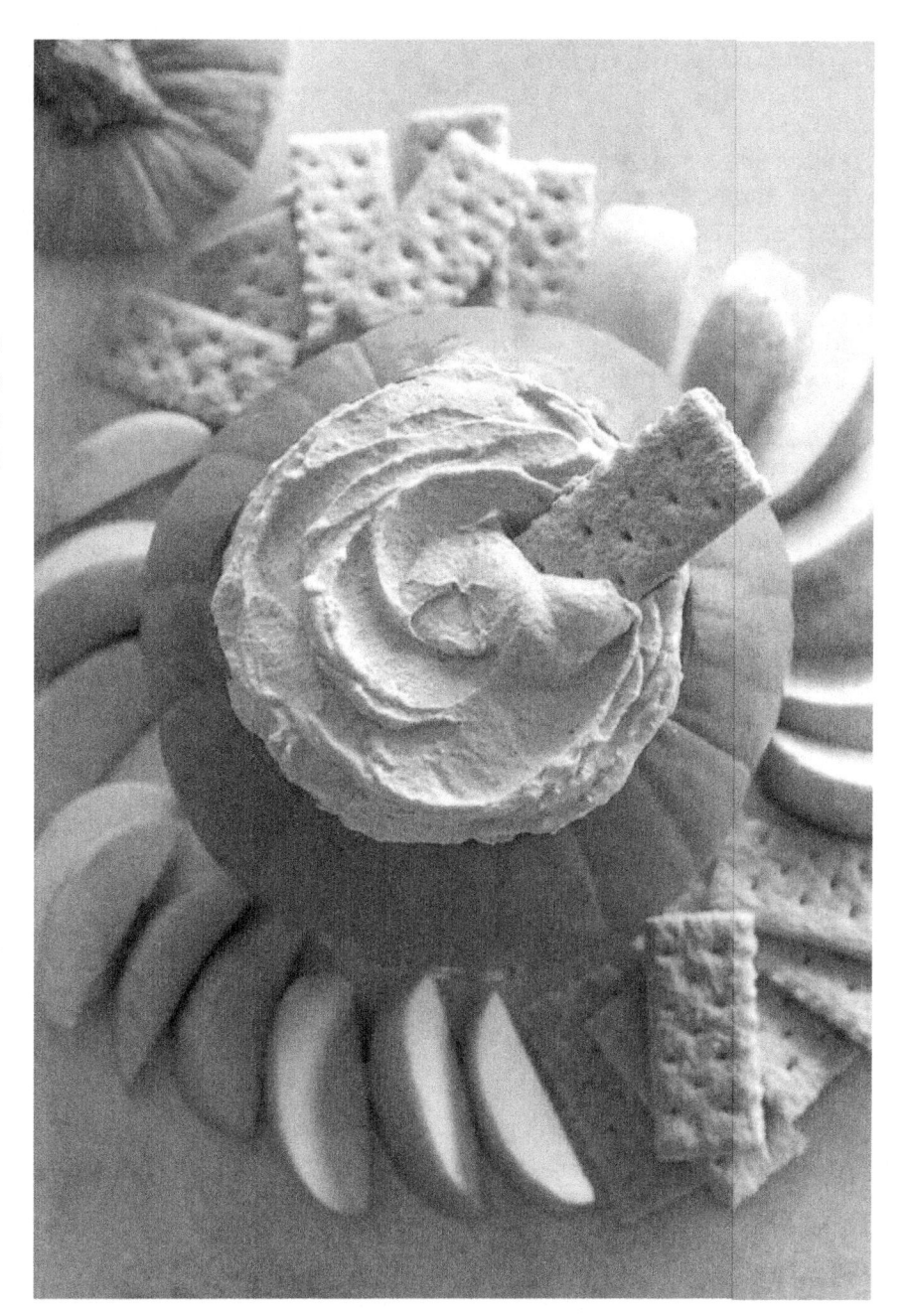

Recipe Notes
1. *You will need 12 oz cream cheese for this recipe (1 ½ blocks) for a nice rich dip. This dip can be made with just 8 oz but will be a little bit lighter in texture and flavor.
2. **One 8 oz container of whipped topping is approximately 3 cups. Measure 2 cups.
3. Beat the cream cheese with a hand mixer for best results.
4. Store leftover dip in an airtight container in the refrigerator for up to 5 days.

NUTRITION FACTS

Calories: 315, Carbohydrates: 38g, Protein: 3g, Fat: 17g, Saturated Fat: 10g, Cholesterol: 47mg, Sodium: 152mg, Potassium: 140mg, Sugar: 36g, Vitamin A: 5350IU, Vitamin C: 1.3mg, Calcium: 63mg, Iron: 0.6mg

Mississippi Sin Dip

PREP TIME: 20 minutes Serves: 12
COOK TIME: 35 minutes
TOTAL TIME: 55 minutes

`14`

The bacon twist on the classic party dip will have everyone coming back for seconds and thirds!

- 1 bread bowl or 1 french bread loaf, or rolls for individual servings
- 8 ounces cream cheese softened
- 16 ounces sour cream
- 2 cups cheddar cheese shredded
- 1 cup bacon crumbles (cooked) about 8 slices
- 1 tablespoon hot sauce
- 2 teaspoons garlic paste
- 1 teaspoon Worcestershire sauce
- ½ teaspoon salt
- ½ teaspoon onion powder
- ¼ teaspoon pepper
- scallions or chives, for garnish

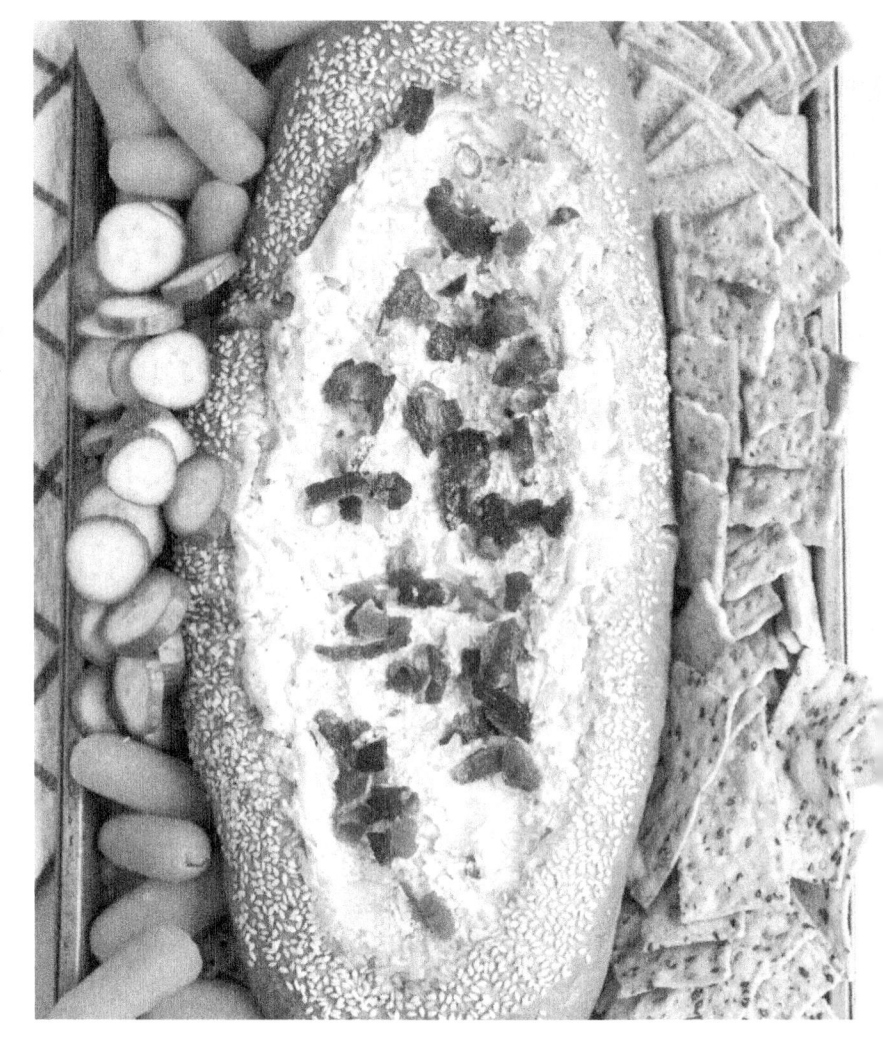

1. Preheat the oven to 350°F.
2. Cream sour cream and cream cheese with a hand mixer until fluffy.
3. Add shredded cheese, cream cheese, bacon, hot sauce, garlic, Worcestershire sauce, and seasonings and mix well.
4. Cut the top off of the bread and remove the insides. Reserve the top and insides for serving.
5. Place the hollowed bread loaf on a baking pan and scoop the cheese mixture into the middle. Bake for 30-35 minutes or until the dip is bubbly and hot.
6. Remove from the oven and rest 5 minutes before serving. Garnish with chives if desired.

Recipe Notes
1. For a milder flavor, swap garlic for ½ teaspoon of garlic powder.
2. When cutting the bread, save the top for dipping. Also use crackers, chips, veggies, and more.
3. Hot sauce can be increased to taste.
4. Mix the cream cheese with a hand mixer. This adds more air to the dip making it more "scoopable".
5. Pre-shredded cheese works well in this recipe (and saves time).
6. Swap out bacon for bacon bits or even sausage crumbles.

NUTRITION FACTS

Calories: 298, Carbohydrates: 3g, Protein: 9g, Fat: 28g, Saturated Fat: 15g, Polyunsaturated Fat: 2g, Monounsaturated Fat: 9g, Trans Fat: 1g, Cholesterol: 73mg, Sodium: 469mg, Potassium: 147mg, Fiber: 1g, Sugar: 2g, Vitamin A: 688IU, Vitamin C: 1mg, Calcium: 200mg, Iron: 1mg

Easy Spinach Dip

PREP TIME: 5 minutes **Serves:** 16
CHILL TIME: 2 hours
TOTAL TIME: 2 hours 5 minutes

| 6 |

A simple creamy spinach dip recipe, perfect for any party!

- 10 ounces frozen chopped spinach 1 package, thawed
- 8 ounces water chestnuts canned, drained
- 2 cups sour cream or Greek yogurt
- 1 cup mayonnaise or dressing, low fat or regular
- 1 package dry vegetable soup mix 1.4 ounces
- 3 green onions chopped

1. Defrost spinach overnight in the fridge or in the microwave. Squeeze dry.
2. Chop water chestnuts and combine all ingredients in a bowl. Mix well.
3. Refrigerate at least 2 hours prior to serving
4. Serve with bread, crackers or vegetables for dipping.

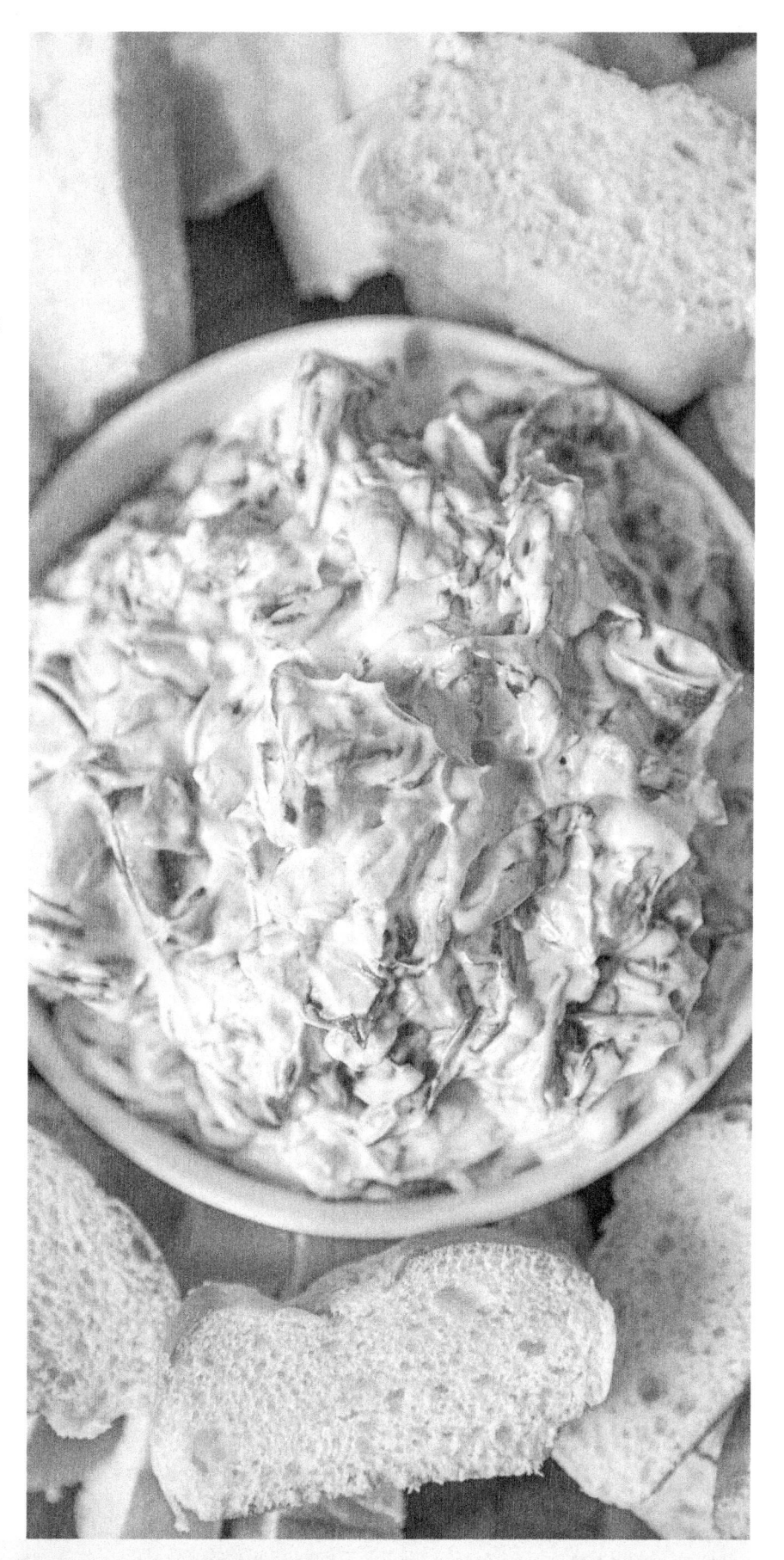

NUTRITION FACTS

Calories: 174, Carbohydrates: 5g, Protein: 1g, Fat: 16g, Saturated Fat: 4g, Cholesterol: 20mg, Sodium: 412mg, Potassium: 153mg, Fiber: 1g, Sugar: 1g, Vitamin A: 2290IU, Vitamin C: 2mg, Calcium: 62mg, Iron: 0.6mg

Hot S'Mores Dip

PREP TIME: 5 minutes Serves: 4
COOK TIME: 1 minute
TOTAL TIME: 6 minutes

15

This is one of the simplest dessert dips to make, it takes just a few minutes & it's so ooey-gooey yummy!

- 1 cup milk chocolate chips
- 2 tablespoons milk
- 2 cups marshmallows divided
- graham crackers for serving

1. Combine chocolate chips, milk and 1 ½ cups of marshmallows in a sauce pan. Heat over medium low and stir until melted and smooth.
2. Pour into an oven safe dish and top with remaining marshmallows.
3. Broil 1 minute or just until marshmallows are lightly toasted.
4. Serve warm with graham crackers.

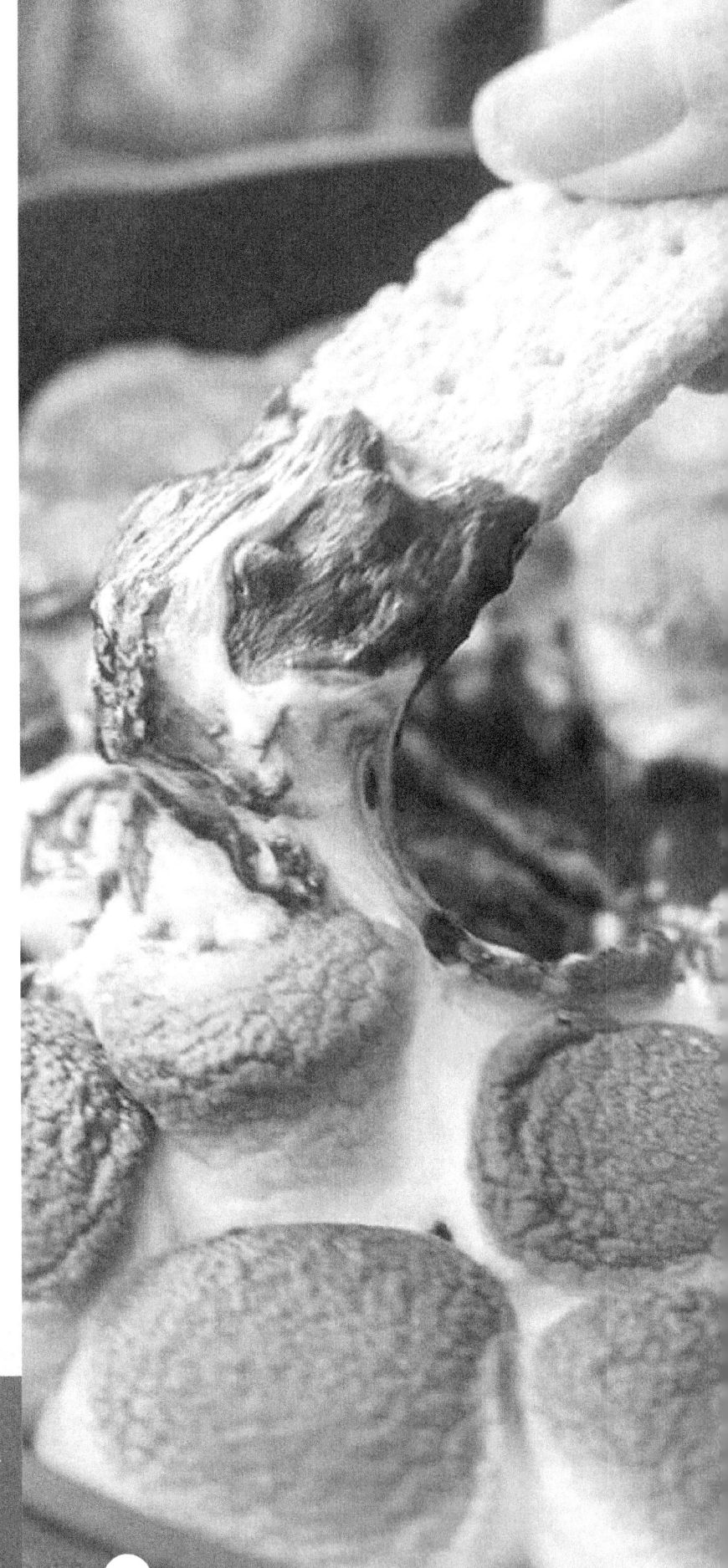

NUTRITION FACTS

Calories: 348, Carbohydrates: 61g, Protein: 3g, Fat: 10g, Saturated Fat: 6g, Cholesterol: 7mg, Sodium: 63mg, Potassium: 11mg, Fiber: 1g, Sugar: 50g, Vitamin A: 115IU, Vitamin C: 0.2mg, Calcium: 62mg, Iron: 0.6mg

Printed in Great Britain
by Amazon